Praise for *Love Your Lady Landscape*:

'Finally someone is writing about the female body, our cycles and our feminine emotional landscapes with wisdom and humour. Lisa Lister brings passion, reality and comprehension to the divine feminine and is making it her mission to educate and create a dialogue that empowers and elevates women to become the modern goddesses we truly are. Every woman needs to read Love Your Lady Landscape *and take back what has been so lost in today's culture.'*
CARRIE-ANNE MOSS, ACTRESS AND FOUNDER OF ANNAPURNALIVING.COM

'I'm a bloody big fan of Lisa Lister. Lead by the Divine Feminine, Lisa is here to write a new story for women and the way the world sees menstruation. Compassionate, current and full of sass, in Love Your Lady Landscape *Lisa guides women to get in flow with their cycle, heal their wombs and reclaim the unstoppable She power that is their birthright.'*
REBECCA CAMPBELL, AUTHOR OF *LIGHT IS THE NEW BLACK* AND *RISE SISTER RISE*.

'Lisa knows the true importance of women loving and honouring their bodies every day. Love Your Lady Landscape *is liberating, fierce and fascinating – and packed with information that ALL women should know.'*
MEL WELLS, AUTHOR OF *THE GODDESS REVOLUTION*

'Lisa Lister is the woman we all wish we were lucky enough to have as our sister. But short of having her on speed dial, this book is the next best thing to a full-on feminine support system!'
KATHLEEN MCGOWAN, ACTIVIST AND INTERNATIONAL BESTSELLING AUTHOR OF *THE EXPECTED ONE* AND *THE BOOK OF LOVE*

'Lisa Lister is sounding the call for you to heal your cycle, accept your ever-changing body and honour your feminine soul. This is the essential foundation and practice for you to get in your 'FLO' and become the powerful force of nature that you are designed to be!'
ALISA VITTI, HORMONAL HEALTH EXPERT AND AUTHOR OF *WOMANCODE*

'Lisa Lister doesn't mess around. She's here to break through boundaries and barriers that have been created, and which society defines as "normal". Teaching and leading women to honour their divinity inside and out is no easy task, and I respect Lisa wholeheartedly. She is part angel, part goddess and part rocker – and her writing is friendly, honest and captivating.'
KYLE GRAY, BESTSELLING AUTHOR OF *ANGEL PRAYERS* AND *WINGS OF FORGIVENESS*

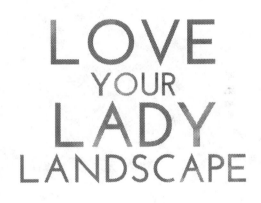

LOVE
YOUR
LADY
LANDSCAPE

Trust Your Gut, Care for 'Down There'
and Reclaim Your Fierce and
Feminine SHE Power

LISA LISTER

HAY HOUSE

Carlsbad, California • New York City
London • Sydney • New Delhi

Published in the United States by: Hay House Inc.: www.hayhouse.com®
Published in Australia by: Hay House Australia Ltd.: www.hayhouse.com.au
Published in the United Kingdom by: Hay House UK Ltd.: www.hayhouse.co.uk
Published in India by: Hay House Publishers India: www.hayhouse.co.in

A catalogue record for this book is available from the British Library.

Interior illustrations: p.90 Lisa Lister/Liron Gilenberg

ISBN: 978-1-4019-6512-9

Printed in the United States of America

I dedicate this book to SHE.

Contents

Contents

Foreword

When you've heard The Call that Lisa describes so powerfully in these pages, a force Lisa aptly calls SHE begins to direct your life. Lisa has helped me realize that SHE has been directing my life ever since I saw my first birth in medical school and dissolved in tears at the wonder of it. It was a holy moment. A turning point in my life. So potent with meaning that I knew I had to become an OB/GYN and sit with women in labour and assist them during birth. It was as easy as breathing.

Thus began my initiation into not only modern obstetrics and gynaecology, but also, alas, into the mind-numbing power trip known as Patriarchy.

I had no words for what I felt at the time of that birth. But I knew in every fibre of my being that this act of womb power was sacred. A powerful portal throbbing with mystery and magic that held the power to transform everyone present. And yet the birthing woman – and her baby – were not being treated with the respect and awe they deserved. And which every instinct in both mother and baby had prepared them for in their first moments of meeting outside the womb. But that's not what happened. Instead the cord was immediately clamped and the baby was whisked off to the nursery to 'clean it up' and make sure it stayed warm. Which it never would have required had it been allowed to stay right on Mom's chest.

The list of these systemic abuses of SHE go on and on and on. Not because people are bad, but because SHE hasn't awakened within them yet. But all that is changing. And rapidly. *Love Your Lady Landscape* to the rescue!

Over the years so much in women's health has cried out to me for healing. I know that I was born to do something about it. And so I have spent decades creating a language of women's health while managing to fit into a patriarchal profession – at least for a while. I have attempted to articulate everything that can go right with a woman's body instead of the approach I was trained in, which consists mostly of cleaning up the devastation of our bodies that results from Patriarchy – the rule of the fathers – in which everything that is feminine and soft must submit to what is hard and masculine.

This is damaging not only to women, but also to the feminine souls of men. And to Mother Earth herself. How else can you possibly explain a culture (at least in the USA) where over 30% of all births are vaginal bypass operations (C-sections), and in which one in three women has a hysterectomy by the age of 60. Can you imagine men putting up with one in three of them having their testicles and prostate removed by the age of 60?

But never mind – all that has been said before. *Love Your Lady Landscape* provides the new path. There are no maps, but there are clues. And Lisa will show you how to recognize them.

This book is the medicine we have ALL been waiting for.

For centuries.

We don't need more diatribes on what is wrong. We already know. It's time to return to the only well that will slack our thirst. To our true source of power. The one we've all been encouraged to forget. And even defile. Because our true power lies in the very places we've been told to be most afraid of. Like our menstrual cycle. Oh – I have to tell you this.

Menstrual blood is the richest source of stem cells known to humanity. Imagine that. Try using some on your plants. Watch what happens. I couldn't resist.

So let's go back to that first birth I witnessed so long ago.

I finally realize, after reading this book, that the altar we should have been kneeling at all along – back then and now – was, and remains, the altar between that birthing woman's legs. And every birthing woman now. Whether we're giving birth to a baby or a book or a garden.

And that is what *Love Your Lady Landscape* is about. How to worship at the altar and the power centre between your legs. Whether or not you've had a hysterectomy. Whether or not you still bleed. Whether or not you have a partner. Whether or not you've had children. No matter what. None of that matters.

Because the power between your legs is always there. Whispering, or screaming, depending upon what's needed.

I've come to see that the practice of modern gynaecology is, after all, largely an attempt to deal with the screaming. So please don't wait until the volume has been turned way up.

Start listening to your precious body now. This book will show you how.

One more thing. You're going to be led, and not by your intellect. That is, after all, how I met Lisa Lister. Our meeting was orchestrated by the Goddess herself. I fulfilled a lifelong dream to take a pilgrimage to Glastonbury, England, last year. I didn't know much about it, and I didn't even realize that Glastonbury is Avalon of the famed *Mists of Avalon* – one of my favourite books of all time. I just know that I was drawn there. On the day we were to visit the

Abbey, this ebullient presence – whom I would come to know as Lisa – appeared across the street with a huge red flower in her lush dark hair, and joy radiating in every direction around her.

Her Viking was on her arm – a guy who is a nurse by training and who shared my medical philosophy. We all hit it off immediately. Lisa led our group to the recently uncovered Magdalene's altar where we prayed and left an offering of roses, and then she took us to a special stone where women sat and bled during their moontime. For centuries.

When we parted, Lisa did something for which I will be forever grateful. She honoured me for breaking trail in this journey back to SHE. And told me how much my work had helped her. Sisterhood. So precious. Nothing like it. We saw each other's souls. We honoured each other. Lisa, like me, has very big ovaries, and a huge heart to match. You need these when you're working for the goddess, 'cause this work is not for the faint of heart.'

I am thrilled to pass the torch to her and her sisters – the cheeky, articulate goddesses who are ready to hold that torch even higher. Unashamed and with great humour, but without taking any bullshit. Let *Love Your Lady Landscape* guide you home. To your pleasure. Your Inner Goddess. And the Power that will never fail or hurt you. Ever again.

Blessed Be.

DR CHRISTIANE NORTHRUP
Author of *Women's Bodies, Women's Wisdom*
and *Goddesses Never Age*

Acknowledgements

Deep bows, high fives and Jem and The Holograms *Truly Outrageous* hot pink lipstick kisses to:

SHE. Always.

My lady landscape – my womb, ovaries and vagina. Teacher, oracle, creatrix and receiver of pleasure. I love you.

The Viking – for daring to join me on my ever-unfolding Lady Landscape adventure despite never knowing where it's going to lead. For holding space as I explore the patriarchy, for holding space as I explore the feminine. For your amazing Friday night nidra classes that were the best writing-a-book medicine, for making me delicious food, for road trips, for loving me, for supporting me, for being my partner in this lifetime. I am blessed to love and be loved by you.

My Mumma – I miss you. I love you. Every day.

Fam Lister – thank you SO much for all your support, love, chocolate-filled care packages and cute nephew hugs and kisses. Blessed to be part of your family.

Team Southsea Coffee – for rawsome Friday morning breakfasts, friendship, nidra sleeps and free Wi-Fi while editing this book – LOVE YOU ALL!

Ani Richardson – for loving, listening, laughing and being so bloody brave and inspiring. ALL the love.

K Dot – you're made of magic, missus, and I'm blessed that you're my friend.

Sarah Durham Wilson – for our boob-out-truth-out calls, laughter and sisterhood. Lady, I love you, thanks for being my sister and friend.

Team Hay House – for believing in this book and me – you rock!

David Wells – for belly laughs, insights, breakfasts and cheerleading. Love you so much astro-dude. Especially when you wear Lycra and shake your pom-poms.

Andrew Stark – for your love, bro-like support and ability to make me cry, snort with laughter *and* source me the most beautiful crystals. I love you.

The SSS – Hollie Holden, Amy Kiberd and Rebecca Campbell – prosecco, spiritual road trips, rituals, cheerleading, the overuse of emojis in every WhatsApp convo and blessed-beyond-measure friendship. Deep bows, morning massages and the biggest love to you gorgeous women!

Aimee Richards-Welton and Sue Rains – for being my BFFs and for knowing me and loving me through it all.

Cat and Leo – for providing a writing locale with rooftop sunshine in Malta – some of my most favourite parts of this book were written in the warm December sun – and for your big, generous, always-sharing hearts.

Maya Hackett – you had me at 'let's be in each others lives forever'. Love you and your vision, woman.

Sephora – for making Jem and The Holograms' *Truly Outrageous* hot pink lipstick. ALL… THE… GRATITUDE…

The SHE Squad – ladies you have the biggest ovaries, thanks for sharing your stories with me. Maria Fanoele, Keeley, Mel Oborn, Stephanie, Silvana Perelli, Lucie, Amy Biondini,

Vanessa @womanspace, Bethany Barrow, Claire Bradford, Jane Caunce, Melonie Syrett, Leanne Lyndsey, Meghan Genge, Nikki Willis, Jocelyn Schade, Kylie Connell, Johanna Meriweather, Georgina Cooper, Laura, Amara Pinnock, Amy Perry, Luna Love, Emma Beal, Naomi Long Srikrotriam, Marleen Smit, Megan McGill, Orlagh Costello, Audrey Meissner, Bronwyn Nash, Sigrid Kleinjans, Ollie Neveu, Katie Hope, Ceryn Rowntree, Tallulah Moonshine, Ebonie Allard, Grace Quantock, Mara Koch, Emily Roberts, Matilda Lundin, Clare Fairhurst, Ali Baker, Kirstie Wilkins, Sarah Starrs, Hannah Lo, Katy King, Cassy Fry, Anna Sansom, Vesna, Vickie Greer, Laura Slowe, Stina Glaas, Jamie Lyn and Lucy Sheridan.

The Call

'You've had the power all along, my dear...'
GLINDA THE GOOD WITCH, *THE WIZARD OF OZ*

There was a time, about 5,000 years ago, when SHE power reigned and lady landscapes were revered.

Temples were built in honour of our curves and statues of goddesses stood 10ft tall. The entrances, shaped like a woman's open legs, were a powerful energy vortex to connect directly with the Divine. It was common knowledge that the womb and belly of a woman housed the power of her badassery: creativity, intuition and manifestation. Yep, the space between a woman's thighs was a power portal, an oracle, a fortune-teller, a direct hook-up to source.

But for over 2,000 years now, our stories, our truths, our wisdom as women have been distorted, censored, burned and unheard. Living in a patriarchy taught us to disregard the potent powers of our wombs. Our connection to Mumma Nature, the lunar cycles and the seasons were ignored, and our menstrual cycle something that was seen as being 'dirty' or 'shameful'.

Now we ignore our root wisdom because we no longer trust that we know ourselves. We look outside ourselves for the answers. We replace creative sensuality with destructive and wounded sexuality. We spend time and money trying to find a new way, a spiritual practice, a community – anything that helps us make sense of ourselves as women, yet nothing fits. When we get emotional or express ourselves fully, we apologize for our tears, suppress our anger and worry that we'll be seen as 'hysterical'. And when THAT happens, we self-medicate with whatever will numb the pain of not being heard – drugs/food/alcohol/shopping [*delete as applicable*].

Worst of all, we have an epidemic of 'down-there' pain and *dis*-ease – pre-menstrual tension (PMT), pre-menstrual syndrome (PMS), polycystic ovaries (PCOS), endometriosis, fibroids and so on. Overwhelm, stress, anxiety and infertility are at an all-time high, while many of us manage our menstrual bleed with synthetic hormones, denying ourselves the experience of living fully in our SHE power.

So high fives, fist bumps and deep bows to you for picking up this book and hearing The Call (you'll read more about The Call on page 21), because hearing it isn't always easy.

Back in 2005, I was living my life from the neck up, operating and making decisions from my head, and completely disconnected from my body wisdom. I worked on a Saturday morning TV show in the UK – the hours were crazy and the lifestyle was fast and fun. I drank lots, barely slept, binge ate in secret, had a loathing for the body I was in and was always trying really hard to 'achieve' the next goal and 'do' the thing that would make people like me/ give me praise/want to sleep with me. (*Ouch. I haven't said that out loud before.*)

Basically, I didn't listen to my gut.

I didn't trust my intuition.

And I definitely didn't feel the feelings.

So it makes total sense that I also didn't recognize any of my body's signals when it was crying out for help. I thought the debilitating period pains, heavy bleeding and rage-full PMT I experienced each month was just a bloody inconvenience. I thought the painful sex and lack of orgasms were part and parcel of being a girl. I made it a mission to ignore the extra 4 stone I was wearing as protective armour by cutting out the labels of my clothes and choosing to wear 'fat, fun and bubbly' as my label instead.

It took what felt like a rather epic scene from Stephen King's *Carrie* where I bled on a friend's sofa, in a quite spectacular and very embarrassing fashion, to finally make me go find out *why* I was bleeding more days than I wasn't each menstrual cycle.

Many months, and misdiagnosis after misdiagnosis later, I was told by a dude in a white coat that I had both polycystic ovary syndrome (PCOS) and endometriosis. His solution? 'Well, as you won't be able to have children, it would make sense for us to just whip everything out.'

It was in that moment that I realized two things:

1. This doctor had zero people skills.

2. I had let others pay more attention to my lady parts (in a manner of interesting and not always respectful ways) than I ever had.

This is when I heard The Call. The Call that has since taken me on an adventure to explore, heal and love my lady landscape. The Call that meant giving up my career as a journalist to devote myself fully to teaching women how to explore, heal and love their lady landscapes too.

The Call that brought you here might not have been a 'down-there' *dis*-ease, it might have been:

- lack of juiciness, sexual desire or passion for life

- miscarriage or termination

- menstrual and menopausal distress

- feeling stressed, anxious or depressed or all three

- anger that your bleed means you're not pregnant – *again*

- overeating or substance abuse to avoid feeling or to fill a void

- feeling uninspired and creatively blocked

- low self-esteem and poor body image

- inability to speak your truth

- reduced intimacy with your partner

- feeling disconnected from yourself, your body, others and/
  or spirit

Or possibly it was one of a gazillion other different variations of how SHE (how I describe *goddess/Divine Feminine/all that is/spirit*) is calling you back into deep and delicious communion with your body: to love your lady landscape, to trust your gut, to care for 'down there' and reclaim your fierce and feminine SHE Power.

Whatever The Call, I'm glad you're here.

You'll notice that the title of this book isn't '*How* to Love Your Lady Landscape', that's because this isn't a 'how to' book – far from it. There isn't a five-point action plan that you have to 'do' in order to reach a final goal, it's not a tongue-in-cheek, car bumper sticker concept nor is it a demand.

**Love Your Lady Landscape is an
invitation for reclamation.**

It's an invitation to reclaim the power of your womb. Our womb isn't just for making babies (which is a pretty badass thing in and of itself). No. When we connect with our womb space (and if your womb has been removed, please know that the womb space itself is still *just* as powerful) and her cyclic nature, we connect with SHE – our all-woman power source. It's where the very best revolutions AND revelations can be dreamed into being.

But you can only begin the reclamation process if you're willing to show up, just as you are – messy, sexual, not sexual, tired, feeling inadequate, scared, excited, sad, angry, hairy legged [*feel free to insert your own feeling of choice here*] and be willing to call back your power.

Y'see it's time.

Our time.

If you're in, then let's pull back the flaps and get intimate with your lady landscape, yeah?

Big love and ovaries,

Lisa x

P.S. When I talk of women and ladykind, I'm referring to women who bleed or who have previously bled but no longer cycle due to menopause or surgically induced menopause. My reason for this is that it's empowering and necessary for us to re-establish our connection to our womb space in terms of her cycles, feminine wisdom and matrilineal power. I acknowledge however that not all women menstruate and not all people who menstruate are women, and I totally welcome a space for opening up the conversation for all those who menstruate, regardless of gender identity. Also, ladykind is very much a word I use as my personal expression of womanhood, if it doesn't work for you, please feel free to replace it with a word that does.

How to Use This Book

I LOVE nothing more than creating a sacred space for women's embodiment, healing, emotional release and creative expression, and *Love Your Lady Landscape* is no exception.

I set an intention for this book's creation under a new moon and then surrendered to the outcome. I visited sacred locations, lit candles, made SHE scents from my favourite essential oils, drank ceremonial cacao elixirs, used master sacraments, painted my nails, danced and moved my body in SHE Flow, had amazing orgasms, walked in nature, was gifted talismans from supportive souls, as the words fell on to the pages of many, many notebooks. (*I write everything in inky red pen on thirsty recycled paper – it's how SHE moves through me best.*)

Don't get me wrong, there *was* a plan, it was a really good one too, but that's *not* the book you're holding in your hands. Why?

**When you work with SHE, the Divine
Feminine, you set an intention
deep in your womb space and then
fully surrender to the outcome.**

It has to start with you, where you're at, right now. You have to let go of any plans or to-do lists or any visions of how you WANT it to be and instead open up your womb, belly and heart to allow yourself to receive your SHE medicine, however and whatever shape and form that takes. This can be tricky when we live in a world where we're taught to set a goal, take action towards the goal and achieve the goal. This a dude-centric concept and one in which a cyclic, ever-unfolding woman (*that's you and me, BTW*) will always feel 'less than' and 'not good enough', which is why it's here that we begin our dance together.

I want reading this book to be a *felt* experience. There's an opening and a closing ceremony and what sits between them is not all set-in-stone factual teachings with scientific proof, most of it is felt, lived and embodied experiences, gathered into three medicine bundles for you.

1. Reclaim Your Lady Landscape

2. Know Your Lady Landscape

3. Love Your Lady Landscape

Each bundle holds:

- **Movement:** SHE Flow practices that will awaken, stir and shake your body to help you to reconnect with, remember and be in total reverence for your lady landscape.

- **Medicine:** Teachings and offerings that will allow you to fully receive and reclaim your SHE power.

- **Muff muses:** The wisdom of teachers, friends, clients and workshop participants who have shared their stories with me for this book.

When I was dreaming into this book, I wanted to cover EVERYTHING.

Everything I share in workshops, classes and retreats. I wanted to talk about the anger, the trauma, the great sex, the bad sex, the fact that we still live in a world where genital mutilation is happening daily – honestly, I didn't want to miss out a single thing, but exploring the blood and guts of being a woman is life-long work and all I really want to do is encourage you to make it a personal-to-you experience, so consider what I've shared as a choose-your-own-lady-landscape-adventure guide, OK?

Also, I have to stress that this book and the work I share in it is NOT linear. There's no plan to follow, there's no right or wrong way of doing things, it's the SHE medicine I've received through reconnecting with my body and her rhythms over and over again – trusting her wisdom and surrendering to her flow – so I can be a full expression of SHE through me and I'm now being called to share it with you.

SHE TRUTH

If you're one of those people who skips the bits in a book where you're asked to contemplate, breathe, move or do a writing prompt, then I'm talking to you. Essentially what I'm sharing in the exercises and prompts throughout the book is *feel-it-in-you-body-ment*, opportunities and invitations to reconnect with *your* body, trust *your* wisdom and surrender to *your* flow and while there's no pressure to write essay-length responses to the prompts or complete ALL the exercises – all I ask is that you're open to the possibility that they will, if you let them, enhance your love-your-lady-landscape experience.

What is SHE Flow?

SHE Flow is a women's movement *AND* a women's movement practice. See what I did there? Throughout the book, I invite you to try a variety of SHE Flow practices and essentially, it's yoga. But it's also *much* more than that.

Now I LOVE yoga but the first time I got on a yoga mat, I cried. At the time I was in a UK size-20 body and for the first time in my life, I felt it move in deliciously different ways. I opened up my hips, I stretched, I breathed and I stretched some more. I can't pretend it was entirely beautiful and serene, but it was the first time my body and I had properly 'hooked up'.

I trained to become a yoga teacher, but soon realized that:

- No matter how much I tried to get my body into certain poses and postures, it just didn't happen. (Or if it did, it felt really uncomfortable and it most definitely wasn't pleasurable, and that made me feel shitty about myself.)

- When I was menstruating my body didn't want to be pulling big-ass warriors, it wanted to be near Mumma Earth in baby pose. (*But I didn't want my teacher to think I was weak so I'd ignore my body, pull the necessary shapes and then feel shitty about myself.*)

- When I was told to hold a pose and 'tuck my tail bone under', my tailbone wouldn't go under and all I actually wanted to do was move my hips like Shakira. (*Except I held the pose, and… you get the picture, right?*)

This is why I created SHE Flow. This *is* your mumma's yoga. It's the yoga of SHE, of Shakti Ma – a delicious and divine, fierce and feminine movement practice that is moon and menstrual-cycle led

– it takes into account that we have boobs, bums, hips and bellies, and allows you to connect fully with your body and to trust that it will let you know exactly what movement it wants and needs.

SHE Flow is inviting and fun, and the nourishing poses don't need to be held for hours – no crazy, pretzel-shape pulling is required and fancy Lycra yoga pants are optional.

In fact, SHE Flow is best done in your favourite pair o' PJs or leggings and 'SHE Flow Yogini' Tee. Y'see, so much of what we know and experience yoga to be in the West is asana-based, structured movement that was created with dudekind in mind, yet it's predominantly practised by women and so often, when we struggle to get our bodies into a pose or hold it for a long period of time, it becomes yet another 'I'm not good enough' stick for us to beat ourselves with. (*And Jeez Louise, we don't need an extra one of those!*)

It's why when practising SHE Flow I encourage you – through movement, breathwork, energy healing and Radical Rest Yoga Nidra (more on that in Part III, see page 210) – to:

- Reconnect with your womb space.

- Come into communion with your body.

- Cultivate SHE, the Divine Feminine, within you.

- Unravel and uncover any repressed emotional energy in your body.

- Listen to your body's cyclic wisdom.

- Surrender to *your* flow.

- Gather your medicine.

- Fully rest and receive.

- Integrate your medicine and then have the big bloody conversations about all that it is to be a woman. ALL… OF… IT…

SHE Flow began as a yogic movement practice to help me connect with my womb and to help her heal. I then mixed yoga with my love of belly and temple dancing, and combined it with the ancient feminine teachings I'd learnt and gathered over the years as a menstrual health and women's wellness practitioner. It now includes:

- womb and yoni massage

- cycle awareness

- self-care techniques like yoni steams and jade eggs

- and medicine-making components, including cacao and shamanic drumming

And so the entire SHE Flow experience was born. I started sharing with small circles of women in my living room and it's now something I'm honoured to be asked to share in classes, programmes and workshops, both online and around the world, and now in the pages of this book with you.

As well as sharing some of my favourite SHE Flow practices with you, I've created a full-length SHE Flow class, and you'll find it along with a digital swag bag of Lady Landscape Tools and downloads at loveyourladylandscape.com

Opening
SHE Ceremony

The air is thick with Lady Nada incense and I am banging my drum to invite you to meet me here, in the pages of this book, to gather your SHE medicine – the teachings and transmissions you most need to love your lady landscape. Not everything that I share will be for you, so take what feels good and leave the rest.

I'm honoured you've chosen me as your guide-ess. Thank you.

A guide-ess is NOT someone who's been there and done it – far from it. She's a teacher *and* a student, a question asker, a provocateur. She holds space for unfurling, witnesses unravelling and offers up signposts for going deeper and/or seeking healing. I will share invitations and conversations but I'm not your teacher, no one's judging you and there's no prize or certificate for reading this book cover to cover or for doing all the practices that I share.

You showed up and you're here. Sometimes that's enough. Sometimes it's not. The chances are though, that you've been called here because you've got to do some freakin' work so:

- Be gentle with yourself.

- Show yourself compassion.

- Be open to receive. Fully.

- Take radical self-responsibility.

- Set intentions, but have no expectations – of me, of the work and, most importantly, of yourself.

∼ Womb breaths ∼

I start every SHE Flow class, every ceremony, every day with womb breaths.

You can do this exercise seated or standing but, if standing, make sure your legs are slightly apart and sink down into your knees to fully allow yourself to connect with Mumma Earth. With each inhale think about what you'd like to invite into your life and with every exhale think of what you'd like to let go of.

1. Place one hand on your heart and the other on your womb space.

2. Take in a deep breath through your nose and let it move through your heart, past your gut and down into your womb (if you don't have a womb, breathe into the womb space) and hold for a count of three. Then slowly exhale, letting the breath pass out through your gut and through your heart, and release fully as an 'ahh' breath through the mouth. Repeat this process as many times as feels good.

3. Now set your intention. Why did you pick up this book? What do you want or most need to receive from reclaiming, exploring and navigating your lady landscape? Make it known now.

4. Take another deep womb breath, place a hand on this book and ask for its contents to be your guide-ess. Ask for it to show you the medicine you, your body and your lady landscape need right now, or set down your own intention in writing – after all this is your ceremony.

~

If you like to be in control and the idea of going with your feminine flow and trusting your body wisdom terrifies you, or your vagina walls are tightening at the mention of your womb as a power portal, then what I share in this book may not always feel comfy.

I'm asking you to be with that uncomfy-ness and simply show up to what you discover in this book with a delicious curiosity. Trust that what feels right for me, might not feel right for you. You may come up against some resistance – in fact, I've worked with enough women in SHE Flow classes, in one-to-one sessions and on retreats to *know* that when talking about lady landscapes, stuff WILL come up. I invite you to witness it, to feel it, to write it down, but not to feel like you have to identify what's 'wrong' or try to 'fix' anything.

That's not the purpose here.

The purpose is to simply get curious about your body, about your womb's cyclic nature and find ways to reconnect with Her in ways that feel juicy, sensual, uplifting and really-bloody-good so you remember and rediscover your SHE power.

You may like to think of cracking open this book like entering into a sacred SHE-led ceremony with your lady landscape. Get still, light a candle, burn some incense or paint your nails red and eat a piece of dark chocolate [*add your own version of ceremonial goodness here*].

Slow your pace, breathe deeply into your belly and womb and, as you read, simply respond to the language of your body and be open to her medicine.

Maybe you'll get visual prompts – you might be out in nature and you'll see a yoni shape in a tree or you'll find a uterus pin badge that you dig, or maybe you'll find a lip colour you want to rename 'SHE Power' because you feel like a badass when you wear it.

Maybe you'll pay attention to that nagging sensation deep in your womb space, the one you've been trying to ignore only to realize that it's SHE trying to wake up in you and maybe, just maybe, you'll enter into a delicious life-long dance with her.

However you choose to express it, I'd love for you to share your lady landscape discoveries and muff musings using the hashtag #loveyourladylandscape on social media, because the more we talk about our experiences, have bloody conversations about periods and discuss our orgasms (or lack of them) over a glass o' red wine with our girlfriends, instead of what's happening with the Kardashians, the less we'll suffer/put up with/keep hidden our pain and womb wounds.

I can't wait to connect with you, hear your stories and be your witness and guide-ess as you begin a lifelong adventure exploring, navigating and, most importantly, learning to love your lady landscape.

PART I

RECLAIM YOUR LADY LANDSCAPE

We are badasses who
make magic with
our pussies.

CHAPTER 1

The Truth Lies
Between Your Thighs

*'There is deep wisdom within our very flesh, if
we can only come to our senses and feel it.'*

ELIZABETH A. BEHNKE

I love my lady landscape.

I love my belly and how the skin has been stretched from 13 to 23 stone and back again, and all the places in between. I love how it's covered in lightning strikes to prove it's a place of power.

I love how I curve at my hip.

I love how my flesh rolls into a chubby Buddha belly.

I love how, thanks to my Romany heritage, I am dark haired and have a lip that needs waxing weekly.

I love that the ink on my skin tells my story in art.

I love my little breasts and their puffy nipples.

I love my clit and her 8,000 nerve endings.

I love my 80s-style bush — which would be frowned on and cringed at by the current wave of shave-her-bare fans.

I love my menstrual cycle (*yep, I really do love it*) and that each month I experience my full cyclic nature as a woman. I also love that during my period I become the epitome of a fortune-teller on Brighton pier. Sometimes I even wear a headscarf and hoop earrings.

I love my womb and how she awoke a calling in me so loud that I now get to talk about vaginas all day. I love that I make fire, creativity and orgasms – the very best lady magic in her.

If I were offered a different body, I wouldn't take it, because this is the body I love.

Just so you know, this is NOT how it has always been.

Learning to love my lady landscape

As a teen girl I had NO love for this body. I hated on it. HARD. My body looked NOTHING like the girls in the magazines that I used to read obsessively.

I was heavy with milky white, almost translucent, skin, slightly spotty and had eyebrows that met in the middle – Frida Kahlo style. I used to wish that my thick, wavy hair were glossy and swishy like 'I'd just stepped out of a salon'. And when I started bleeding from my vagina each month and growing inordinate amounts of hair on my upper lip, under my arms and 'down there', I declared to anyone who would listen, 'You may as well shoot me now, because being a girl, in THIS body, sucks.' (*Yes, my drama-queen tendencies started at a young age.*)

This hate–hate relationship with my body didn't get any better in my early 20s. In fact it got worse, as I studied and entered the industry that was responsible for so much of the hate in the first place – glossy magazines – ironic, don't you think? Luckily for me though, I got a job with *Just Seventeen*. This magazine was different to the others. I'd grown up reading it – it was kooky and fun. It used real girls as models and reading it was like being part of the best girl gang ever. Unfortunately, along with lots of teen magazines at the time, it folded a few months later, and I found myself entering the harsher 'shiny' world of TV and glossies.

SHE TRUTH

Full immersion into the world of shiny hair and perfect lip-lined pouts is NOT recommended if you lack the self-love. Just saying.

Every interview with a size 8, midriff-bearing new-on-the-scene pop star made my self-worth shrink and my waistline grow. From the outside, my life looked pretty peachy – I was meeting pop stars, writing for magazines, travelling and partying – a lot.

Except when I got home and shut the door, I'd eat ALL... THE... THINGS...

Why?

I felt like a fraud. I was fat in a world of thinness and eating became my tried-and-tested method of self-medication and, as for the whole bleeding from the vagina thing, it took on new levels of suck.

At the time, I was living with a dude I thought was my forever-love. We were engaged and had a mortgage. It was all thoroughly grown up. But I was bleeding more days than not each month. Supposed-to-be-my-forever-love found this annoying because it meant we had less sex and he liked sex.

Surprisingly, I found it annoying because it felt like my womb was being ripped open by a chainsaw over and over again, and the heavy-duty sanitary pads that always lined my knickers were all that stood between me being known as the one-woman projectile bleeder. Seriously, I bled on office furniture, on friends' sofas, straight through a white dress when interviewing a new five-piece boy band. (*Luckily their PR girl took pity on me and helped a sister out by giving me the heads up before I hit the streets of London.*)

Eventually my bleeding became so embarrassing that I went freelance so I didn't have to leave the house. I got a reputation as a total flake amongst my social circle because I'd say yes to going out and then cancel because I was bleeding – usually with an industrial sized hot water bottle strapped to my belly and high on painkillers.

The medical profession were less than helpful and offered me birth control to 'manage' the symptoms. The bleeding and pain were bad enough but being on the pill drove me bat shit crazy and on more than one occasion saw me threaten supposed-to-be-forever-love with the gouging out of his eyes with a spoon. (*In retrospect perhaps funny but at the time scary because I totally would of have done it if he hadn't been so cat-like on his toes.*)

Then, after two or three years of trying various different drugs and misdiagnosis after misdiagnosis, a dude in a white coat did lots of tests, poked and prodded my 'down there' a lot and called me back to his office.

I asked supposed-to-be-my-forever-love if he'd come with me because, well… I had access to Google and I'd pretty much self-diagnosed myself with death-by-vaginal-bleeding but predictably, he was busy so I went solo.

As I shared earlier (see page xxi), the test results showed polycystic ovary syndrome and acute endometriosis. I had no idea what any of those words meant, but finally they had a name for the thing that I had – two names, in fact… This was good news, right? They'd be able to do something about it, right? Wrong. Less than 10 minutes later I was outside the doctor's office revelling in the newfound knowledge that my womb was also called a uterus (why had I never been told that before?) and holding a leaflet describing the procedure to remove it and all the bits attached to it.

One sheet of A5 paper was the total extent of information they could give a woman about removing her ENTIRE reproductive system.

WTF?!

I took a long walk home because I had some stuff to figure out. The supposed-to-be-my-forever-love and I hadn't even discussed the possibility of children and now I'd just been told that I couldn't have them. Forget the supposed-to-be-my-forever-love, I hadn't even thought about whether I wanted children or not and now that possibility had been taken away from me.

My womb, also known as my uterus, hurt. Not from the nagging pain I'd grown accustomed to feeling over the last few years, but a different pain. It was a fist-shaking, 'I'm angry' pain. It's what I now know to be SHE, the Divine Feminine, awakening in me. At the time though, I didn't know that. I liked crystals and did spells at the full moon, but I'd never thought – not for one moment – that a fierce and feminine energy in my womb was moving through me and shouting, 'Wake up, woman. Connect with your body, trust yourself – this is not OK!'

I sensed it though.

I sensed it when I got home and, after explaining the situation to the supposed-to-be-forever-love, he said, 'OK, so after you have the operation, we'll be able to have more sex, right?'

I sensed it a few days later, when the leaflet from the doctor remained unread on the kitchen table and I signed up to a goddess retreat in Glastonbury and didn't entirely know why.

I sensed it when I read *Eat, Pray, Love* from cover to cover and realized that a pile of bricks, a mortgage and a supposed-to-be-forever-love were simply not enough – that I was worth far more than that. *Elizabeth Gilbert, I heart you.*

If you've read my books *SASSY* or *Code Red*, you'll know that supposed-to-be-forever-love, was NOT my forever love. No surprises there, right? What followed was a lot of chocolate-eating and gin-drinking, a lot of feeling sorry for myself, a lot of sleeping with people I probably shouldn't have to make myself feel loved and validated, and a lot of arguing with supposed-to-be-forever-love about money and piles of bricks.

What followed after THAT is when the story *really* began.

Getting curious about 'down there'

Just so you know, I call it 'down there' with my tongue firmly in my cheek because doing the work I do, I talk about vaginas/pussies/ muffs/vulvas/minges/cunts/yonis ALL DAY. (*But can you believe there is still no one word that we can call our own when talking about our lady landscape? Let's add that to the list of things we need to have a bloody conversation about and underline it five times, yeah?*)

It felt like the pain, the discomfort, the fact that I had to leave my job and the fact that the supposed-to-be-forever-love turned out to be a douchebag, was actually SHE, via my labia lips, communicating with me.

SHE didn't want me to have sex or be in a relationship with someone who didn't love and support me when life got a little shitty.

SHE didn't want me to be doing work that made me feel bad about myself.

And most of all, SHE was clawing at me from the inside, desperately wanting me to reconnect with my body, with my womb, and heal her, so that I could help heal other women, because ladies, we're in this together.

**When we heal ourselves, that
gaping big gash of a bloody wound
we're all collectively walking
around with slowly starts to heal
– literally and metaphorically.**

Yep, I had a pissed-off vagina, and there's a good chance you have, too.

Why?

We've been given the forget-that-you-are-powerful drug, along with, conveniently, the forget-that-everything-you-need-is-already-inside-you drug. Basically, we've been anaesthetized to our own pussy and our power by the patriarchy so that we are easier to control and manipulate.

And it's worked.

REALLY... BLOODY... WELL...

Her story

There was a time when the female body was seen as a living embodiment of Mumma Earth. Like her, SHE experienced cycles and seasons, not just within a year or a lifetime, but every 28 days.

We've been taught that the only purpose of our monthly cycle is for a woman to become pregnant, but that's not true. During the time it takes the moon to circle the Earth, we give birth to life, we cultivate life, we make sure life is fertile and we allow life to die.

And then we do it all again.

**We experience a whole life cycle,
the whole SHE bang, EVERY...
FREAKIN'... MONTH...**

That right there, is bloody lady magic, but there's more... Each phase of the menstrual cycle also represents a phase of a woman's life:

- pre-ovulation – the maiden

- ovulation – the mumma, the creatrix

- pre-menstruation – the wild and wise woman

- menstruation – the elder, the crone

And in each cycle, during each phase, we're able to gain teachings and a deeper understanding of, and from, that particular archetype.

While many of us have been taught that our bleed or 'time of the month' is a curse, indigenous people around the world know that it holds a super-sacred role in that when a woman bleeds she not only sheds an unfertilized egg, but also the unfulfilled dreams, pain and emotion of that cycle. Not just for herself, but also for her entire family and community.

For that reason women once gathered in red tents and moon lodges, and refrained from doing their daily chores because they were doing epic and powerful transformation and purification magic with their wombs – not because they were 'dirty' or 'unclean'.

Towards the end of the bleeding time, once the cleansing has taken place, her intuitive powers are super-strong. She is able to create a direct hook-up to SHE, the Divine Mumma and receive creative ideas, transmissions, wisdom and insight for herself, her family and her community.

**Lady magic is the VERY best
kind of magic. Fact.**

SHE TRUTH

This is happening in you, and me and every woman who bleeds. We have the power to detox, cleanse and heal our entire body, our emotions AND those of our family and communities every time we bleed.

I know, right? We are badasses who make magic with our pussies.

Our powers were seen as way more potent than just physical strength, and were a direct reflection of Mumma Nature. The Great Mumma called us to celebrate all the gifts that the feminine and female body offered: the ability to create life, to cleanse, transform, manifest and purify, to connect with source and a heightened intuition, and to completely accept the necessity of the cycles of life, birth and death. When we did, we knew that the light we saw was simply another vaginal opening birthing us into our next human experience because we knew we were eternal.

We were fearless in the face of death because we experienced it each and every month when we bled.

RARRR!

Is it any wonder dudekind got scared and fearful? That they did all they could to disconnect us from our bodies and our power source? And felt the need to suppress and contain the feminine?

I blame patriarchy

Now before you call me a patriarchy pummeler, we need to be clear about a few things. Patriarchy is a male-dominated power structure in which men have power over women and that is NOT OK. Not one little bit.

It's NOT, however, a term I use to blame men for everything. I love dudes (especially hairy ones with beards), so when I talk about patriarchy, I'm talking about the constructs and the structures, not ACTUAL dudes.

I blame patriarchy for pulling the plug on our insta-connection to source.

I blame patriarchy for rebranding the teachings of Jesus. (JC was totally Team Woman. He and Mary Magdalene taught the way of love, honoured the feminine and respected the female temple arts and teachings of Isis, I'm certain of that. Sadly his PR team, a patriarchal boy squad, did a great job of spin-doctoring his teachings.)

They cast Eve out of the Garden of Eden to create a sense of universal rejection among ladykind, made Mary Magdalene a prostitute and banished Lilith to the place of myth and legend.

They made it so that we needed a spiritual go-between when we connected with source; they made that spiritual go-between a dude, and totally dismissed our Great Mumma – despite the fact she'd been worshipped for thousands of years previously – and they made that source our father.

I blame patriarchy for creating a new way to experience time that no longer reflected or honoured the cycles of the season.

I blame patriarchy for doing everything it could so that women no longer recognized their reflection in Mumma Nature, and now, thousands of years later, we no longer recognize our reflection AT ALL.

I blame patriarchy for how, generation after generation, women have slowly become reprogrammed and repatterned to either act like a dude or to please a dude.

I blame patriarchy for making mothers and daughters testify against each other during the witch trials. Declaring that the prosecution and persecution of witches – which, if you're not familiar with it, was the term given to wise women and healers – was being done in the name of the mother church, which created womb-deep mistrust amongst women and a totally messed up story of sisterhood that is still prevalent today.

I blame patriarchy for why we deny ourselves our own pleasure, urges, needs and desires. Why we mistrust our own inner wisdom and guidance. Why we deny ourselves connection to source and in so doing, deny ourselves our power.

Yep, I blame patriarchy for ALL of that.

A note about the dudes

When I read this to the Viking (my husband) his initial reaction was, 'Wow… do you think it's a bit much?'

Now, the Viking is a dude who's awake. He's a force for feminine good, and he supports, loves, worships and honours the Divine Feminine and the work we do together in our relationship with each other (*and it's definitely work*) to navigate the union of the masculine and feminine. He nurtures, agitates, inspires and grows me on a daily basis, so this was *not* the reaction I was expecting.

I was rage-full when I wrote it. I was also pre-menstrual. The two are not mutually exclusive. I chose to write this section in this phase of my cycle (you'll find out more about each cycle phase and its super powers in Chapter 4), so that I was in my full pussy-to-the-earth truth. It was conscious anger and I dared to feel the fire of carrying over 2,000 years of my ancestors' anger and grief at being a woman in my womb and ovaries so, yes, I was pissed and guess what? I make no apologies for that.

I was pissed at patriarchy and, if I'm honest, I was pissed at the Viking because I thought he'd be like, 'Hell yeah, sister! Preach!' But he's been anaesthetized too, we all have, men AND women, and while he definitely doesn't fear a woman in her power, he's still very much learning to navigate the experience and what that means for him as a dude in the world, because the masculine is wounded, too.

So be gentle with the dudes. Unless, like me, you're also in your pre-menstrual phase, in which case shout a few obscenities, slam a door and play Taylor Swift really loud.

Seriously, for most of us, knowing, respecting and loving our lady landscapes is still uncharted territory, so expecting the dudes to have a full understanding of our entire female experience and become a fully signed-up member of Team Woman is definitely an ask. Not a *big* ask, but it's still an ask. Just like us, they've got a lot of unpicking and unschooling to do of what they thought was truth, too.

Patriarchy has done a job on us.
On all of us, men AND women.

Women perpetuate patriarchy as well. I was in a room a year ago with some of the most impressive-on-paper women, leaders in their fields. I was excited to spend time with them but so disappointed when, what should have been a big-hearted, open discussion, turned into what felt like a my-penis-is-bigger-than-yours conversation.

Most of my clients are women with busy lives and have no other point of reference than to lead from their dude energy. They've disconnected from their bodies so that they can keep 'doing and achieving'. They wear game faces to cover their crazy-painful PMT, have no time for a relationship and use stimulants so that they can use every hour available in the day to 'keep up'. This constant pressure to perform and be wonder women activates a continuous stream of competition and comparison with other women – 'She's had a baby, she's got her figure back and she's back to work in four weeks – I hate her!'

But the chances are that woman hates herself, too. Ladies, we don't need to grow a pair of balls, we need to grow a vagina. One of my favourite quotes is from *Golden Girl*, where Betty White said,

**'Balls are weak and sensitive. If you
wanna be tough, grow a vagina.
Those things can take a pounding.'**

Hell yeah, Betty!

When we know better, we do better – Maya Angelou, esteemed poet and civil rights activist, said so. So get to know your lady landscape intimately – the collective and the personal wounds, your wants, desires and urges, your cyclical nature. Connect with SHE on every level – physically, emotionally and spiritually through your womb space. Then share what you discover with the dudes in your life, and ask them – if you want to, of course – to join you in the exploration. It's not always easy, as the Viking will testify, but we need to call dudekind *in* and stop calling them out.

It's in the darkness we grow roots

The patriarchal anaesthetic is industrial strength and is perpetuated by men and women every single day. In the advertisements we see, in the magazines we read, in the language we use.

It's why women are:

- Shaming/manipulating/calling out other women daily.

- Doing all they can to 'hold it together'.

- In a constant state of comparison and not feeling worthy.

It's also why at 25 I hated myself, couldn't keep up with my fast-paced life, self-medicated with food, and didn't know that a womb and a uterus were the same thing until a dude in a white coat threatened to 'whip it out'.

The patriarchy had put all my power in the darkness and taught me, rather successfully, to be scared of the dark. Yep, all the parts of being a woman, all the keys that enable us to access our power in this lifetime – our menstrual cycle, our pleasure and desires – have been hidden in the shadows and labelled taboo, so that it's too bloody scary for us to go there, discover them and claim them as our own.

Well, 'til now that is.

I'm a Scorpio and I'm not afraid of the dark and nor should you be, as it is in the darkness that we truly grow our roots.

Deep roots.

Roots that provide stability and safety.

Roots that provide a bullshit filter to the concepts of competition and comparison of being less than and not enough.

Roots that provide the strength to own ALL the parts of you.

Strong roots.

Roots that make it harder to be manipulated by advertising and the media.

Roots that make it harder to believe that playing small is a career choice.

Roots that make it harder to be mocked, taken advantage of, shamed and blamed.

Fierce roots.

Roots that mean you'll dare to be visible and seen.

Roots that mean you call forward revolutions and revelations.

Roots that mean you'll call out bullshit.

Connected roots.

Roots that reconnect you to the natural cycles of Mumma Earth.

Roots that reconnect you to your cyclic, ever unfolding and unfurling powers.

Roots that connect you to your truth.

Powerful roots.

Roots that remind you to never ask permission.

Roots that remind you that SHE is you and you are SHE.

Roots that remind you it's not a race, it's a journey.

**When we grow roots, we take
back our power and we rise –
grounded and full-bodied.**

∼ ROOT BREATH ∼

To help grow strong and firm roots, the root breath uses *Mula Bandha*, meaning 'root lock'.

This yogic practice combines muscle contraction and energy stimulation to turn energy in your root chakra located at your genitals (for more on the chakras see page 180), into creativity and healing energy for your entire body. Don't practise root lock breathing during menstruation.

1. Take in a deep breath through your nose, hold the breath and contract your anus. Feel the muscles lift upwards and inwards.

2. Keep these muscles contracted and then contract the area around the vagina. You'll experience a slight lift, as you do when trying to stop the flow of urine.

3. Now contract your lower abdominal muscles and pull your belly button towards your spine.

4. Apply these three actions together in a smooth, rapid and flowing motion (don't worry, it make take you a few practices to grasp!) and allow the energy to travel up your spine and out through the top of your head.

5. Exhale through your nose.

6. Repeat the root lock as many times as feels good, some people do five, others 25, but it's most beneficial when practised daily. Go slow with it and gradually allow your muscles to strengthen and the movement to become smoother. You might like to try a set of womb breaths (see page xxxii) each morning followed by 10 root breaths.

CHAPTER 2

SHE Power

*'Mine is just a simple old human story – of one
person trying, with great rigor and discipline, to
comprehend her personal relationship with divinity.'*
ELIZABETH GILBERT

So basically, I started to love my lady landscape when a voice in my womb, which I now refer to as SHE, started flapping her labia lips at me.

I am TOTALLY aware of how freaky-deaky and woo-woo that sounds. Before then I'd never connected to my body, not really. In fact, if my body could have told you it's story, it would have gone a li'l something like this:

*'I've always been a 'big girl' body and that has
embarrassed Lisa and made her feel the need apologize
for it. She thinks we take up too much space – there's
too much of us. She thinks that she's a completely
separate entity from me. Our relationship sucks.'*

It's true. My body and I simply didn't get along.

So it's a rather comical plot twist that it took the diagnosis of 'down-there' diseases and a labia lip-flapping source of power that resides in my womb space, to hook us up.

As a teen girl, I had no love-yourself guidebook, I'm guessing you didn't either, none of us did, but what I know now that I didn't know then is that you don't need a guidebook. None of us do – the map, the guidebook, the blueprint as to how to be a woman is in our freakin' womb.

We were bloody born with it already inside us.

Except no one told us.

No one told our mummas either. Or if they did, very few of them knew how to articulate it to us.

Now, I'm not going to keep pointing the finger but patriarchy – just so you know – I AM giving you an indefinite side-eye, which is why this book, and everything I share in it, is one big arrow-pointing-towards-your-crotch sticky-note reminder.

My womb is my power source.

Repeat it a few times; roll it around your tongue. Say it out loud. Whisper it. Feel where it lands or meets resistance in your body as you say it.

It's a truth.

It's THE truth.

Yet, it might not feel entirely comfortable, not yet. In fact, it might feel like you can't handle it or don't want to handle it and that's OK. The only reason I know it to be true is because I've FELT it and until it is a felt experience in YOUR body, it'll have as much meaning to you personally as a meme being shared on social media.

When we're told daily that our body is a commodity and that it needs to be cut, nipped, tucked or starved in order to meet an unrealistic, airbrushed ideal of so-called perfection, how do we begin to feel that truth? How do we begin to feel that the space between our thighs – the space that for so many holds so much blame and shame, hurt and trauma – is our source of power? How do we feel anything at all when we've become comfortably numb from the neck down?

Slowly.

This is a journey, not a race. It's an invitation to set out on a lifelong exploration of your lady landscape. Just so you know, when most people go on an adventure, they pack a bag full of things they may or may not need, but when you go on a lady landscape adventure, what you'll find is that there's a lot of UNpacking to do.

Uncovering your stories, thought patterns, beliefs and false truths – not just your own, but those of family members and friends, those of your culture and the society in which you live – I'm not going to lie, is big freakin' work and, no pressure, but you're doing it on behalf of *every* woman that has ever been and *every* woman that is to come. The good news is, that the work – and when I say work I mean work of the very best kind – pelvic-deep healing, play, pleasure and joy – starts and ends with you. When you do the healing work for yourself, you WILL heal ladykind.

Our starting positions won't be the same, our terrain – physically and metaphorically – will be different, but our reason for showing up?

Ah, now that is the same for each and every one of us.

Lady, you've been called.

Called Girl

So, I promised you earlier that I'd talk about The Call and that's because I'm a Called Girl. (Not to be confused with a *call girl*.

That's something entirely different. Although, if you're not following your big beat-y heart and you're pimping yo'self out in a job or a life you don't dig, there might be something in that.)

A Called Girl experiences life, moment to moment. She's in tune with the feminine cycles, rhythms and seasons that allow her to fully own her divine, feminine SHE power. She works in, not out. She trusts herself and thoroughly enjoys inhabiting a female body.

A Called Girl knows that self-acceptance has to come before self-improvement.

A Called Girl doesn't hold on too tightly to a defined and specific outcome. Instead she shows up, roots into Mumma Earth, listens to her pussy, trusts her gut, raises her heart and boobs to the sun and remains open to the infinite possibilities that occur when you collaborate with SHE.

Sounds good, right? But what if…

You fuck up?

It doesn't turn out how you expected?

Or…

It goes really freakin' well and you feel overwhelmed?

Let the fear and anxiety be there, and do it anyway.

Do it without any concern as to what it might be or how it might turn out, or what it might lead to, but simply because you've been 'called'.

I dare you.

Looking back, I can see that SHE left clues for me throughout my childhood and her biggest one was a cartoon character – She-Ra. My idol. I'd watch *She-Ra: Princess of Power* every week and her story went something like this:

She was captured as a baby and held captive by a mind-controlling force. *(Since birth, a mind-controlling force – patriarchy – has captured us ALL.)*

She's gifted a sword of power by a sorceress to lead the Great Rebellion against the mind-controlling force. *(We've ALL got access to a power source and when we recognize it in the root of our female body, ladykind will no longer be so easy to manipulate and control.)*

She calls on her allies with special powers to battle against the mind-controlling force. *(Our allies are each other and when we connect with our bodies and heal ourselves, our power becomes strong and we no longer need to compete and compare and instead we are able to help and support each other.)*

She consults with a higher power for guidance in a crisis. *(When we connect with SHE, we're connecting with a force that is in us and is also bigger than us and SHE has our back. Always.)*

She was largely non-violent and would only use combat as a last resort. *(You don't need to be violent when you can shoot lightening bolts of SHE Power from your vagina – metaphorically obviously.)*

Basically She-Ra showed me the story of ladykind's reclamation and when she pointed that sword to the sky at the end of every episode, it was my call to action.

Except, I was eight and eating toast and jam.

SHE called me a few times from the age of eight until the threat of the 'womb whip out'. For sure, it was subtle – more of a labia-lipped whisper than a full vaginal shout, but I chose not to hear her, because being a Called Girl takes ovaries. It means daring to undo everything that you have so far believed to be true. It means identifying habits and behaviours that are keeping you numb because you're too scared to feel.

Feeling is a super power. Fact.

It means looking at your relationship with yourself, your family and culture because how you currently perceive and experience these will be a direct reflection of how you perceive and experience your SHE power.

So yep, for a long time I opted for the comfier I'll-stay-just-as-I-am-thanks option.

SHE TRUTH

This option doesn't stay comfy for long. SHE may let you off when you're eight, but if SHE feels that SHE's being ignored, SHE will turn Kali Ma (the dark goddess) on your ass and make you dance like your vagina is on fire. If SHE's ignored for too long, SHE will call you to burn it all down, discard what you think you know, and scream and claw at you until you listen. This is my experience of Her. Your experience might be different. In fact you'll probably hope and pray that it is, but honestly? I'd wish for nothing different.

Let me introduce you to SHE.

SHE is the Divine, the Great Mumma, goddess, priestess, healer, witch, wise woman, wild woman, shamana, spiritual homegirl, bitch. SHE is every feminine archetype you know, as well as all those you are yet to discover.

SHE is me and SHE is you.

SHE is your gut instinct.

SHE's those times when you dance like no one is watching and SHE's those times when you dance like EVERYONE is watching.

SHE is messy, wild and untamable.

SHE encourages you to come undone – over and over again.

SHE takes you to the dark because she knows you can handle it.

SHE will encourage you to destroy and let go of the parts of yourself or your life that no longer serve you.

SHE wants you to rise, of course SHE does, but she wants you to have strong roots, too.

SHE gives meaning to your voice.

SHE is unbrandable.

Her guidance – your intuition and inner knowing – resides in your belly and womb space and is incredibly accurate and so, through knowing SHE, you become both vulnerable and fearless in claiming your power, no matter what.

**SHE shows up without an invitation
and demands that you do, too.**

SHE was kicked to the dirt and pushed underground by the patriarchy and grew strong because, despite what patriarchy will have us believe, the feminine is NOT afraid of the dark. In fact, it's where she does her best work because she IS the dark.

It's why, if you're experiencing a 'down-there' *dis*-ease, if PMT is all-consuming, if you feel like you're being kicked in the vag by depression, anxiety, fear or life in general, I urge you to look down.

I urge you to take a big deep breath in through your nose, all the way down to your womb space, hold it there for a moment or two, release the breath through your mouth and drop down.

Come IN to your body, come into your womb space and meet SHE there.

SHE's been expecting you.

~ BODY CHECK ~

You can't just rest into an intellectual and/or heart understanding of this work, you need to feel it in your body. Except we're desperate to get out of our bodies – we want to escape this human experience – but this invitation is completely the opposite, it's calling you *in*.

I invite you, each morning before getting out of bed, to connect with your body and check in. Enjoy being IN your body. Rub yourself, rub your belly and tell your womb, 'I love you.' Check out what's going on in your womb – create a hands-on-your-flesh relationship with her. It's essential and fundamental.

It's so simple that your mind and ego will rage against it. Your mind wants everything to be complex: it wants answers, it wants to complicate things. Get familiar with simple.

Everything I share is intended to be felt not intellectualized and so, if in doubt, place a hand on your womb space, breathe deeply and check in with your body. Your body is your home, so keep coming back to her.

~

Connecting with SHE

As I was dreaming into what this book would be about, I read lots about Malta's prehistory and Her sacred lady landscape. This little island just below Sicily, Italy, is the epicentre of SHE, and over 50 goddess temples and womb tombs over 5,000 years old grace her landscape. I heard The Call and I booked a flight. Just so you know, it's now my favourite place in the world.

One hot afternoon the Viking and I visited Hagar Qim and Mnajdra, two of the biggest, temples on the west side of the island. As we entered the sacred site, a guide – a small and smiley Maltese man – waved his hand and called me over to him. I smiled and obliged. (The Viking is used to this, as I am somewhat of a hit with the over 50s). The guide, dropped his smile, placed a hand on mine and told me in a super hushed and serious tone, 'You are the *Maltese Dreamer*, you are here to do the work of SHE.'

Fo' real.

I got the full body chills, a sure sign that sacred shit is about to go down.

(If you don't know the *Maltese Dreamer*, it's a statue of a sleeping big-hipped goddess that was found in the Hypogeum, an underground womb tomb in Malta.)

The guide, or *my* guide as I now call him, sat with us for over an hour talking about the temples and how no one speaks to their feminine prehistory – the official literature questions whether the 7ft-goddess statues found at Hagar Qim were in fact sumo wrestlers. (*I know, right?!*) He spoke about how they were a place of goddess worship and how their main purpose was to draw down the power of the stars into the womb of the Earth.

My guide shared a ritual with me that he instructed me to do in the first chamber of the Mnajdra Temple. He said that I'd be alone and that SHE would welcome me there. Looking around me, the place was full of tourists, but my guide assured me it would be fine, as he ushered the Viking and I on to the coastal path down the cliff towards Mnajdra. At the temple entrance, the crowd dispersed, and I was alone in the first chamber, just as my guide had predicted.

I whispered the incantation he had given me, stood with my legs hip-width apart and took in some big deep womb breaths (see page xxxii). I began to feel roots grow up from the earth, from the bones of all the women that had gone before me and worshipped, prayed and bled on this land and I felt loved, I felt strong and I felt in my power because I knew SHE was me and I was SHE.

I was connected directly to source, through my body. I wasn't looking outside myself to a higher power, I was rooted deep into Mumma Earth, the ground under which the goddess had been driven by patriarchy. I felt the stories of the ancients, my blood and bone, run through me, begging to be told in a time when they'd truly be felt and heard, and I felt home.

Listen with your womb

You may recognize Her voice as your own. You may not. It may come from a deeper place or sound more authoritative, or more loving, or stronger than the voice you use in everyday life. You may hear nothing. You may want to punch your meditation cushion in frustration, but keep showing up. Keep asking questions, keep breathing and staying open to receive.

SHE makes herself known when I write in my journal, so I have a gorgeous red leather journal dedicated to SHE where I riff, without editing, every single day. I set a timer for 25 minutes and let myself write uninterrupted. I write anything and everything to clear any nonsense and allow SHE to speak through the written word.

You could also use tarot cards and oracle sets, too. I use the SASSY SHE oracle cards, a divination tool that I created under the light of 13 full moons and they are the many faces, guises and aspects of SHE. Each card has a one-word prompt that can act as an icebreaker between you and SHE when opening up communication with her.

∼ SET UP AN ALTAR OR
A SACRED SPACE ∼

Set up a sacred space in your home that is just for you and SHE.

Take in a deep breath and ask for SHE to show herself to you. What colours, sensations, textures, images, music appear?

You may need to do this a few times but SHE will guide you and send you signs – collect images, textures and female power icons that call to you.

Make the space as sacred and fun and as beautiful as you'd like. Add anything that makes it more personal to you and SHE – a candle, some flowers, incense and so on. Tend to your sacred space every day and add more items as you feel called.

You may choose to sit and write, breathe, meditate or chant here each morning, let it be your touch point.

If you're short on space, you can make a mini portable altar in a small tin with a lid (for example an Altoids tin) or make an online altar using Pinterest – both are great ways to access SHE.

∼

Trust SHE

This is the hard bit. SHE wants to speak to you, really SHE does, but you're probably so used to the super-loud voice of doubt, not being good enough and feeling inadequate being played on a consistent loop in your head, that it might be hard for you to trust that a loving, attentive, fierce and feminine power source wants to support you and help you heal. But this is the work. It's lifelong, and the more you do, the more you'll uncover. The more you show up for yourself, the more you'll be able to trust that when you trust SHE, you trust you. When you know SHE, you know you. And that's when you can really access your SHE power.

When I talk about SHE power, I'm not talking about the kind of power that involves wearing 80s-style shoulder pads and blue eye shadow all the way up to an over-plucked brow. No, I'm talking about your incredible, deliciously divine, fiercely feminine power.

SHE Power is the wisdom of your ancestors, your g-mummas and their g-mummas before them. The wisdom of all the wise women that have gone before us – Isis, Astara, Kali Ma, Mary Magdalene, Joan Jett, Boudicca, Joan of Arc, Cleopatra, Maya Angelou, the Black Madonna, Sheena Na Gig, Lalita Devi, Akhilanda.

SHE power is your wisdom. It's burning fire, it's Shakti (feminine energy) that's held in your cauldron, your womb, your entire pelvic bowl, and released with each and every menstrual cycle.

It's ancient, it's powerful, it's magic and it's potent.

It's your intuition – your divine knowing.

It's your body's own inner GPS system.

It's the good stuff – the bloody good stuff. (*Pun totally intended.*)

But being called to reclaim your power and rise, be seen and express yourself is really bloody scary, particularly if you've been completely disconnected from the roots of femininity.

We live in a society with no guidance or structure for the female experience. We're told that in order to 'achieve' and 'succeed' we have to 'do' life like a dude. Advertisements for menstrual products tell us not to let our 'time of the month' stop us from 'taking on the world', and movies and pornography have become the barometer for how our genitals should look and how we should be having sex. Yet so many of us are either experiencing a no-desire zone or we lack the ovaries to ask for what it is we *really* want/need/deserve. Is it any wonder we have no recollection of our SHE power when we've been completely disconnected from it?

Your SHE power simply needs to be reawakened, owned and stepped into.

Now, when I say simply, I don't mean easily. There are no shortcuts.

You still have to show up for life's assignments. In fact, you'll have to face them head, heart and womb on. You have to really feel them in your entire body because where they show up and how they make you feel physically, is a clue as to what they're trying to teach you. Then, and only then, can you release your old way of being and step into your SHE power.

Basically, there's no room for playing small.

You have to surrender to a new possibility.

A new perception.

The newness and total vastness of this may feel a little scary, but don't go mistaking scary for exciting.

Exciting is good.

Rediscovering your SHE power

And it *is* a case of *re*discovering, because honestly, you've had it all along, it's always been there – INSIDE YOUR WOMB.

Yep, meet SHE within your beautiful, imperfectly messy you-ness rather than looking outside yourself for the answers and you will always, always, always find the truth. Any neediness you may experience in every day life will lessen and your insecurity will weaken.

But you have to be willing to go there.

Now, I've been working with my SHE power for over a decade, but that doesn't mean for one moment that I've got it totally figured out. As I've been writing this book, BIG questions have come up for me about my experiences as a woman, an author, a wife, a potential mumma, a businesswoman, a lover and all the other titles we're offered up.

It's been an interesting time.

SHE TRUTH

Interesting is code for messy, emotional, heart-hurt-y' with lots of swearing and shouting. Just so you know.

It has stirred a puddle of dark fears and rage that had been lying dormant at the bottom of what, on the surface, looked pretty clear. When that happens, you have a choice.

1. Get yogic and observe the ripples; watch as the shit rises to the top – fears, concerns, anxiety – and acknowledge that you are not the fears, concerns or anxiety.

Or

2. Sack off all you've ever learnt in a yoga class or self-help book and dive pussy-first into the muddy puddle and have it out with the Divine.

What can I say? I love a good mud wrestle.

The Viking took cover as the moon waxed and waned, and waxed and waned over again, as I wrestled, hugged, loved and cried with Kali Ma in search of my truth of what it means to be a woman – this woman.

No matter what any guru/author/teacher may tell you, it's totally necessary to get down and dirty with the grit of being a woman, yet so many of us are afraid to go there. We're worried by what might happen if we allow ourselves to feel rage, anger and grief in every fibre of our being for as long as we need to.

We don't dare to descend. We're fearful of poking around in the darker and difficult parts of our personalities.

Yet the whole point of descent is to work through our shit, integrate what we learn and rise happier and wiser and a little bit more awesome than we were before. It's the heroine's journey – the ancient story of the Goddess Inanna.

It is the female initiation. Except, ancient female rites and rituals have been replaced with saccharine-sweet tales of happily ever after and back-to-back episodes of the Kardashians because we live in a culture where emotion is often labelled as 'dangerous', 'crazy', 'hysterical' or 'irrational' – so we put as much distance between ourselves and what we feel as we possibly can.

We find our favourite ways to numb out. (*Mine is sugar and reality TV.*)

We push down the dark stuff because we're told to 'think positively'.

We go off looking for ourselves in therapy, in exotic locales, in relationships with totally inappropriate people we know are no good for us, carrying designer handbags and wearing pretty shoes.

And we wonder who we are.

We turn down our light and are nice and likeable. We're told that if we express ourselves fully by shouting, screaming and climaxing, we're wild and uncontrollable. In the words of Isadora Duncan:

'You were wild once here.
Don't let them tame you.'

But the truth is, we *have* been tamed. We're heavy with the shame and guilt carried by our lineage. It's why we talk about periods and sex and pleasure in hushed tones. It's why we don't trust our own gut. It's why we rely on the media to dictate how we think and feel about others and ourselves. It's why we numb our pain with excessive food, drugs or alcohol. It's why we compete with our sisters and feel resentment and animosity when their life – played out through pictures on Instagram/Facebook/Twitter – looks better than ours.

One thing I know for sure is that at the bottom of each of our puddles, there is an underlying rage — which belongs to our mumma, our g-mumma, our gg-mumma – and it needs to be stirred, felt, experienced and expressed.

Now, I totally get non-attachment and that by rolling in the mud I'm going to make messy handprints all over the whitewashed walls on the way to spiritual enlightenment, but what my mud wrestles with Kali teach me each time and time again is that I need to fully experience being this woman — the pain, the anger, the joy, the pleasure, the mess, the dirt.

I am woman, and I WILL freakin' roar.

I will also cry. I will scream really loudly during sex and not give a shit what the neighbours think. I will take time off when I bleed each month. I will run my business in total sync with the moon and my menstrual cycle. I will fully feel and express the rage of my lineage.

I dare you to feel it.

I dare you to experience it.

I dare you to express it.

Unapologetically.

Get down and dirty with the grit of being you.

Invite Kali Ma to play – she plays rough but it's with the love of the great mumma – and dare to go there. From that place then go on to create, love, start a business, have sex, write a book, dance, sing, travel. The world is missing women who are willing to live life belly-deep in the mud and grit of what it really is to be a woman.

How do you know when you've connected with your SHE power?

You'll feel connected and fully in your power. You'll breathe slowly. You'll feel nourished and full up, regardless of what's going on in your external world, and exude a confidence that comes straight from your core, the kind that simply cannot be manufactured.

Not living your truth, not connecting with your SHE power, looks and feels a lot like this:

- Comparing yourself to others.

- Bitching or complaining.

- Trying to be something you're not.

- Frantic, anxious or overwhelmed.

- Bingeing on food, alcohol, drugs, your social media stream or TV as a coping mechanism.

This will show up differently for each of us, but knowing the difference between the two will help you to know when you're aligned with your SHE power and when you're not.

For example, if I take on a new project or meet a new person my litmus test is to ask, 'How I am breathing, what do I feel?'

This awareness of your deepest feeling is the key to staying on your truth path. And you've got to dig the truth path. So to awaken the powerful SHE power that's eager to come through you:

- Be aware of when you're out of whack with your truth.

- How you act, talk, think, and breathe when you're not in alignment with your truth.

- Pay close attention to the differences in how you feel.

Know that by paying close attention, things *will* start to change and that seeing things differently is the Kali Ma catalyst for spiritual shifts.

These shifts can sometimes be a 'bit' uncomfortable (*Ha! that's a total freakin' understatement*), but that's a good thing.

Every experience, scenario or person you meet is a powerful opportunity for you to strengthen your SHE muscle. Repeat the mantra '*I am willing to know my truth*' and trust that SHE will guide you.

Feel your truth.

Allow your SHE power to pass through you, to guide you and energize you to experience a newfound self-awareness. Basically, SHE is asking you to unlearn everything you've been taught to be true about yourself by the masculine paradigm.

Think less and feel more.

This is the new story.

This is the story that I'm rewriting because the one we've been led to believe as being truth about women is in fact bullshit.

The story where we are 'too much' or 'not enough'.

The story where we forget to dance, to touch ourselves, to undulate in our own pleasure.

The story where we don't come into deep and juicy communion with the Divine, with SHE.

The story where we ignore our wild, untamed and cyclical nature.

The story we are not celebrated at menarche, don't honour our menstrual bleed time, and instead curse it and wish it didn't exist.

The story where we have no idea who the fuck we are because we don't dare, or know how to claim and stand in our SHE power.

THIS is why I'm here.

It's my mission to make talking about our wombs, ovaries, vaginas and cyclic nature less science-y and more relevant to our daily life so that when a doctor suggests a 'total whip out' or you blame yourself for breaking, not conceiving, thinking you're going mad or feeling depressed, you'll know why and what to do about it, and you'll also be able to help a sister out if she's in a similar situ.

I want girlfriends to be discussing periods, hormones, pain, anger, sensuality and what they desire over a glass of red wine while eating dark chocolate and having a yoni steam (see page 216).

I want us to never have to feel like talking about our lady parts is TMI.

I want us to have ways to understand and deal with a dry vagina, low sex drive or a lack of desire.

But I cannot do it alone.

It needs ALL our voices.

Your Call may be packaged differently, you may not be called, like me, to write books that include lines like 'shooting lighting bolts of SHE Power from your vagina', but whatever job title you may give yourself – PR assistant, Mumma, consultant, burlesque dancer, HR manager, wife, dog walker, lover, yoga teacher, editor, caregiver – we are ALL being asked to retell the story of SHE.

Chapter 3

Feel It to Heal It

'Nothing in life is to be feared, it is only to be understood. Now is the time to understand more, so that we may fear less.'

Marie Curie

What is your current relationship with your lady parts?

The potent fierce and feminine SHE power, held in the cauldron of a woman's body — her pelvis — is the very energy that is most needed in our world at this time. When I asked the gorgeous women in the SHE coven — an online circle I hold space for — what their relationship with their lady parts was like, I was inundated with responses:

'I hate the pain every month that almost makes me sick and radiates down to my knees. The heavy clot-ridden periods that make me wonder if something is wrong. Knowing very well I should have had a child by now or at least an 'accident'. Wondering if I can have children and hoping I can because now I actually want them.'

'She does me proud. She gives and receives mind-blowing pleasure and gave birth to my beautiful son, yet, if I'm really honest, she's looking a little old and messy.'

'I love my lady parts but I need to heal the way I have learned that vaginas are ugly and disgusting. For a long time I thought there must be something wrong with me because my flaps were too big or my clit was wrong. I think vaginas need a voice to share that they are beautiful in all shapes and sizes.'

'It's a work in progress. I had two biopsies done on my cervix and I haven't reached up to see how it feels since. I don't want to know what it feels like now, I want it back the way it was. I'm told by my doctor that I'll eventually need a hysterectomy and I don't want it really, I can't imagine not having a period.'

'Trying to reassure my lady-bits that the perimenopause doesn't mean the end of ladyhood.'

'Mixed. I am slowly accepting that I am a woman and not a man, and there are things that I can't/won't do now to honour my lady parts. Treating them gently and caring for them is my next step. Even sex is a bit of an effort right now – my lady parts want to be treated to an orgasm every now and again but it's hard to do this through penetrative sex, so I tend to ignore them in favour of my husband's pleasure and I get mine where I can.'

'I feel disconnected. I am pregnant and it is now constantly leaking, which is normal but annoying. I have NO sex drive at all and my partner is a little freaked out about pregnant sex, so we haven't been connecting regularly and I am a bit worried it won't be the same after giving birth but I just don't really ever have that desire I feel like I have always had. I can't see down there anymore, it's very difficult to trim up and I am worried that I will rip down there during birth. I am trying to show it love and send good thoughts down there.'

*'It's not too fantastic on the whole. I have days where things
are better than others, but when my womb decides to go
nuclear on me and cause me pain and general misery,
it's difficult to find the love. The days where I feel in tune
with my cycle and my body are epic. I feel invincible and
that's just amazing. But on the whole, it's not great.'*

I can talk about how powerful and awesome it is to be in your body
as a woman. I can talk about your womb space as a power portal,
but if you've suffered a prolapse, if you bleed more days than you
don't each menstrual cycle, if you're in a relationship where you
daren't ask for what YOU want, if you've been raped, experienced
trauma, had a hysterectomy, have painful fibroids or one of the
other hundreds of different 'down-there' dis-eases, me telling you
to love your lady landscape is going to make both you and your
lady parts pretty pissed.

So what's *your* relationship with your lady parts?

There's no judgement, no right or wrong response. I'm simply
asking that you check in with where you're at, right now, in relation
to 'down there'. Just be open to what she does or doesn't say.

If you need a little kick-start, 'womb love' is my non-negotiable
daily practice for coming into connection and relationship with
your lady parts.

~ WOMB LOVE ~

Use this really simple connection technique every morning to
connect to your lady parts. Doing this daily will help you to own
and operate from your creative SHE power generating centre,
and recognize the most sacred aspect of who you are.

Read through the instructions below then begin.

1. Take a deep breath and close your eyes.

2. Energy flows where intention goes so bring your attention directly to your pelvic bowl and create a yoni mudra. (Mudra is an energy lock you create with your hands.) Put your hands out in front of you, palms facing down, place the tips of your thumbs and first fingers together to create a diamond shape and place it below your navel on your womb space in total reverence and love for her.) Big sigh.

3. Be with her. Hold her. Thank her.

4. Tell her, 'Uterus, you rock!' or 'I think you're bloody brilliant' or 'I love you, let's be wombies' – or make up your own love notes to your womb and share them using the hashtag #loveyourladylandscape – I want to make a sticker set!

5. Notice how your womb space literally starts to pulse and light up (this may not happen the first time you do it, but be patient with her), as the nitrous oxide (NOX) – the endothelial lining of the blood vessels – creates blood flow in your womb space. NOX is the distillation of our body's feel-good juice, its life force, its rocket fuel – basically it's the REALLY good stuff. If you do no other exercise in this book, please for the love of SHE, do this one.

6. Send her love.

7. When you feel like your connection practice has come to an end – mine can vary from a 5-minute check-in before I hit the shower, to a 30-minute love-in, lying on a sheepskin rug in front of my altar chanting to her and sending her love – bring your hands into prayer at your heart.

This practice will be easier on some days than others – especially if your womb has been holding on to trauma or anger for a long time. If you're not feeling the love, if you're angry, if you're mad, if you're teary – I ask you to stay with those feelings for as long as you can and really feel them. Your feelings are facts so they can – and will if you let them – provide you with the medicine that you need.

~

Trust your medicine

When I talk about medicine I'm not talking about the type dispensed at the pharmacy counter, but the medicine that we gather throughout our life to help us to learn and grow.

My nanna (the most awesome gypsy witch you could ever have met) taught me how to work with plants and herbs as teachers, to make feel-better potions and tinctures, how to use the energy of the moon cycles and the seasons to plant and how to change state so that I was able to access my intuition more deeply. She also taught me that 'this too shall pass' when someone else's words cut me deep. But most importantly, what she taught me was that medicine rarely comes from the bathroom cabinet; medicine comes from Mumma Nature: experiences, words and feelings.

Except, seduced by chocolate, boy bands, bad men, a career and consumables, I forgot. Perhaps you've forgotten, too.

We can make our own medicine.

For me, movement is medicine. Ceremony and ritual are medicine. Cacao is medicine. Womb wisdom is medicine. Yoni steams are medicine. Menstruation is medicine. They're all ways that help me integrate and understand what I'm learning in this lifetime.

Through reconnecting and remembering, through exploring my lady landscape and through my work with clients, I've cultivated a deep and thorough practice of listening, dedication, surrender and responsibility, which I believe is essential when working with womb medicine.

I hope that's what you are nurturing in you right now.

I hope that you're beginning to trust yourself and your inner wisdom.

To listen deeply to what feels right, and what feels wrong in your body.

To recognize the cosmic winks when they appear and to follow them and surrender to them fully.

And above all, to take personal responsibility for ALL... OF... IT...

SHE TRUTH

It may feel safer for you to work with a practitioner or therapist while exploring the practices and experiences that I share.

We've been numb for too long and we need to feel. We need to feel in order to heal.

Healing the female wound

Every time we sense a patriarchal pattern in our being – when we worry about our waistline, when we're told that we're not OK and believe it, when we compare ourselves to another woman, when we think that we are undeserving, not good enough, that we need to play small or one of the many, hold on too tightly to an outcome or any other patterns that we let define our everyday experience as a woman – admit the truth.

Admit EVERYTHING because truth and integrity can happen when we keep admitting to everything.

Admit it all without fearing judgement. Admit that despite everything you've learnt, you need to be reminded over and over a-freakin'-gain that the world needs what you've got.

Admit to it and we blow it up.

My friend Annu Tara says, 'Be Her Revelation.' Don't you just love that? I'm going to get it tattooed.

Reappropriate the tools that perpetuate these patterns – social media, for example. What if you didn't stick to the rules? What if you dropped the buzzwords and memes and simply let your social media feed become a story, something that honours your needs and your voice and your ever-changing nature?

What if you didn't have to be just one thing? What if your 'brand' or 'social media feed' became a raw, ever-expanding expression of who you are? For example, I post on Instagram almost daily because I love it. I don't post on Twitter because I don't love it. I don't have a separate feed for my business and for me because I'm not separate from anything. If we're going to embrace the wholeness of who we are, let's drop the masks. Let's show up, just as we are.

For me that involves wearing hot pink lipstick one day and talking about 80s cartoon characters the next; talking about the power of cacao as a shamanic plant teacher and sharing my PMT rage about the way we are ravaging Mumma Earth because I am ALL... OF... THESE... THINGS...

Consistency is an illusion. Ladies, we are cyclic and we've been boxed in and told to create, perform and act within restrictive linear boundaries for far too long. Feel all the expressions of SHE in you throughout your menstrual month, feel them fully and let that become your guiding force.

This is SHE power in action.

Be vulnerable.

Witness what's yours and what's definitely NOT yours. Act accordingly.

Trust yourself, trust SHE and let YOUR labia lips do the talking.

Feel SHE in your body in a glorious, shameless, confident, luminous way. Go inwards and connect directly to the collective wisdom of the sacred feminine that has always been there and comes through every woman, as she listens to the whisper/scream/shouts/cries of her womb. When you do, it will return you – and us – to the essence of being a woman – all that is free, wild, intuitive, natural, cyclical, alive and fiercely loving.

The Mumma story

Except, it's really hard to be a fierce and feminine container of SHE power if we haven't addressed the places within us where we've felt banished, abandoned and disconnected from Her.

I know that until I heard my labia lips flap for the first time, the concept of the goddess was a laminated picture of Kali Ma on my altar. I loved her like I love Frida Kahlo and Cleopatra – as a badass woman I was completely separate from.

I worshipped Kali through prayer and gave her offerings at the turn of each season, but she was very much a deity I dug from a distance. Obviously I now know her intimately, we mud wrestle when shit gets real, but there was a time when SHE and I were not one of the same. That's because our first encounter with SHE/the Goddess/the Divine Feminine is our first encounter with our mumma, so until we have the courage to 'go there' with our own mumma story, SHE will remain simply a picture of a goddess on an altar, a fairy-tale concept of how things might have been.

My relationship with my mumma was… tempestuous.

I craved love and attention and was constantly looking to her for approval. My mumma came from a family of eight and married a man in need of constant attention. Inevitably she fought for attention within her family and, more than anything, she wanted to be loved and cared for, too.

And so it begins.

Neither of us were having our needs met. My story was her story and her story was her mumma's story.

Then when I was 13 my mumma left home, leaving me to look after my dad while she declared that she'd fallen in love for the first time, that she had never been so happy; and I didn't hear from her for four years.

I felt abandoned, unseen, unloved, not validated and rejected.

I now know these wounds to be one of the reasons that I ate (consistently) through my teen years. I needed to numb the pain of rejection and being unloved by the one person whose approval I wanted the most. It's the reason I've worn fat like a suit of armour because I couldn't bear the pain of anyone hurting me again. It was some pretty grizzly and painful work, but it was fundamental in setting me free.

Our mumma provides our template for how to be a woman in the world. Bethany Webster writes about this so powerfully in her blog post 'Why it's crucial to heal the mother wound' at womboflight.com. So any limiting patterns and beliefs that we might experience through that original relationship with our mumma – consciously or unconsciously – become internalized as our truth. The way our mumma treated herself is the way she treated us and this becomes how we think about ourselves deep in our core.

In the same way that dudes aren't entirely to blame for patriarchy, our mumma isn't entirely to blame for our experience either. Mummas are human. They have flaws, just like me and you. So when they pass down beliefs like 'stay small, it's safer that way' or 'don't use your voice' or 'don't stand out' – while they may be well-intentioned and well-meaning, these messages are holding us back from being able to live fully in our SHE power.

The good news is that whatever you've inherited from your mumma doesn't have to be your destiny. Hurrah. You CAN transform what you've previously believed to be true. After a lot of 'going there', I was able to thank my mumma for showing me that family patterns *can* be changed. She dared to follow her heart – no matter what the consequences. She dared to fill her emotional well first – to put her own needs before mine – by doing so, she was able to share her love with me fully in the years before her death.

SO… FREAKIN'… POWERFUL…

The pain of being a woman in this culture has been passed down through generations so when you work to heal your mumma story, you begin to transform and heal the collective female story. You heal the women that have gone before you, and the women who are yet to come.

I am high fiving, deep bowing and sending you the big love for THAT.

In those first days, weeks and months of your life, you and your mumma are tight. You are one of the same. So whatever stories and wounds your mumma was carrying, in those early days and moments of your life, those stories and wounds became your stories and wounds.

Owning our SHE power means that we need to reflect on our mumma story. It holds so much information about where we came from, why we're the way we are and how we've become tangled in these patterns.

Your relationship with your mumma is one of the biggest keys to self-knowledge.

Your circumstances, situations and experiences will be different to mine – maybe your mum drank and wasn't there for you; maybe she was overprotective; maybe she worked so hard you never saw her; maybe she left you at birth; maybe she didn't know how to show affection – there are a million different variations of this, and no fingers need to be pointed. We just have to deconstruct the story before we can rewrite a new one.

Do you feel like you're keeping yourself small because it makes you feel safe? Do you feel like your life has been on hold because you're waiting for your mumma's permission to claim your own life? Do you fear that your mumma will feel threatened, if you shine? Do you have a pattern of emotional caretaking? Do you need approval? Do you worry that your mumma struggled and sacrificed so much for you that you'd be abandoning her if you succeeded?

What I've found from my own experience and coaching clients over the years is that the biggest mumma wound for so many women is that we just don't feel safe. It's in our bones and it was in our mumma's bones and her mumma's bones to be scared. They burned us for being healers, witches and heretics – of course we're scared. But becoming witness to your mumma story and the wounds that come with it, can begin to make it safe, because they're ready to be seen.

They're so ready.

Be your own mumma

My mumma left her body at a time when society, my body clock, my friends, the Viking's parents were calling me loudly to become a baby-mumma.

I'm not sure if my body is capable of baby making and I'm not sure that, even if it were, I'd want to but what I *am* sure of is why my mumma left her body at this time.

It was a call from SHE to trust my own mumma instinct to be real, raw and bold in the world.

I love and miss my mumma every day, and it's in her death that I'm receiving SO many teachings from her about our relationship and who I am as a woman, most of which would just not have been possible for us to do in real time.

Our relationship with our mumma is intrinsic to our relationship with who we are as a woman. If your maternal needs weren't met as a child, it will have a MASSIVE impact on your story. Your self-esteem, your ability to show love to yourself and others, your sense of worth are all dictated by how your mumma was able to show you love when you were a young girl and how you were celebrated (or in most cases not) at menarche – our first bleed, our initiation into womanhood.

This is the story of EVERY woman – and I don't want to trivialize it by speaking about it briefly – but I invite you to explore the relationship you have with your mumma and how she, or the maternal figures in your life, have influenced, shaped and defined the story of you.

This relationship impacts your ability to tell your own story, too. If, as a child when you spoke, you were told you were silly, the chances are you may have difficulties speaking out now.

If you didn't receive what you perceived as enough love and hugs, you may not believe that what you have to say matters or deserves to be heard. FYI: It absolutely does. Just saying.

It's blocks like these that can stop us from really living our story, from being our own leading lady and from sharing our badassery with the world. It's why, if you've read *Code Red*, you'll know that I'm passionate about hosting Red Reconnection ceremonies for women. These ceremonies allow a woman to return to her menarche, to step back into the body of herself as a young girl and meet herself there. Fully. It's a really potent and for some, life changing process (see Resources, page 247).

It wasn't until I revisited my own menarche story that I realized I hadn't been heard or listened to. I was ignored by my mumma at that moment of my first bleed and told it wasn't important, so that set the tone for the relationship I was to have with myself as a woman and my ability to speak and share in the world.

It's why I articulate myself better through the written word. When I speak in public, the words sometimes get jumbled and my voice shakes. I do it anyway, because *I* matter – my story matters.

The good news is that we get to rewrite the story and throw ourselves a menarche party (see page 123) or a Red Reconnection ceremony at any age. We get to be the one who gives that girl who's becoming a woman exactly what she needs.

Whether your mumma is still on the Earth plane or not, it's important that you become your own mother, that you recognize and take responsibility for meeting your own needs, and more importantly that you know your needs are worthy of being met.

Your mumma medicine

There isn't a fill-in-the-blanks exercise to find your mumma story and simply fix it, and I don't expect for one minute that doing the exercise that follows will be all the work you'll ever need to do either. I went to see a therapist weekly for three months to help me get to the point where I could see my wounds, how I was self-medicating them, and why and how it was effecting my ability, or lack thereof, to show up fully in the world as a woman. I still go every six months to keep cleaning up any new discoveries so I can be as clear a vessel as possible. I also have yearly hugs from Amma. Some call her 'the hugging saint', I simply call her 'Ma'.

Amma is the living embodiment of love.

When my mumma died, Amma was my guide-ess. She says, 'An unbroken stream of love flows from me towards all beings in the universe. This love is my inborn nature.'

To be embraced by Amma is how I imagine it is to be curled up in the cosmic womb where there is only love, compassion, selflessness and good. I also say prayers to Ma Devi at my altar each morning, I call her into every class I take and every ritual and ceremony I share, basically I do the work every day.

The following practices will help you to scratch the surface of what is true to you. When you connect with your relationship with your mumma – and what you went through as a child – you'll find it easier to empathize with yourself and give your inner child (*I totally balked at that phrase for so long, so I get it if you do too!*) the mothering she needs to feel safe again. As we create an inner bond of safety, we can really feel our roots begin to strengthen. The deep roots that allow us to stand strong in our SHE power, to be successful, to be visible, to mess up and to speak our truth.

This version of you, the flawed, messy one who shows up and tells her truth is what the world is waiting for. So many of us have had to wear a mask to survive, it's time now to drop the mask and to trust that you matter and that your story matters. Oh, and in case you didn't know, I think you're awesome.

∼ Exploring your mumma story ∼

Download the SHE Flow class (see page 247) and move with the questions that follow.

Sweat, scream, cry and pray out the answers. Feel them IN your body and then crack open to a clean page of your journal and let your womb, gut and heart collide with pen and paper. (You can type if that feels good for you, but I really think there's a different kind of power when you write by hand.)

All of the journal prompts below are best accessed by moving your body but how you process and explore what comes up is your call. Write a poem or song, draw or make art that represents the feelings. Express what comes through in a way that feels real and true to you.

- What is/was your relationship with your mumma?

- What was it like as a child?

- What is your menarche story? Can you go back to that time of your first bleed and remember how you felt, what was said, how your parents reacted? (*This may take a little doing, because for so many of us this was such a non-event that we've pushed it aside, but try to go there, heart riff it out without editing and then try to tap into the emotions that you feel as you experience the story – are you sad, are you angry? Are you embarrassed?*)

- How did your mumma show you love?

- How do you show love to yourself and others? (*When I talk about self-love, I'm not talking about a nice bath – although that's obviously delicious, especially with pomegranate and rose bath oil – but the fierce love that means you're able to say no, set boundaries, know what your needs are and make sure your needs are met, be unapologetic – THAT kind o' self love.*)

- What are your needs? And are you able to be your own mother? (*This is a biggie, so be gentle with yourself and don't be afraid to reach out for help either. You may want to seek the support of a councillor or therapist in your local area. Take responsibility for what you need and know that I love you, a lot.*)

~

Once we begin to process the pain of our mumma story, the pain no longer needs to stay in the darkness where it manifests as manipulation, competition with other women and self-hatred. Our pain can be felt, experienced and hopefully, over time, turned into love – a love that reveals itself as fierce support of one another and deep, radical self-acceptance, freeing us all up to be fully in our SHE power. *RARRR!*

~ **Mantra to the mumma:** **Vishwa Shakti Avaham** ~

I use this mantra every morning as part of my daily connection practice to SHE. I use my mala beads (a string of 108 beads with one bead as the head bead called a *Sumeru*, which are used as a tool to help the mind focus on meditation, or count mantras in sets of 108 repetitions) and then chant the following mantra (pronounced *vish-wah-shuck-tee-arrva-hum*) 108 times.

'Vishwa Shakti Avaham'

I use this mantra to connect to my womb because it connects us through our matriarchal line back to the original creation point of all things – the womb of SHE, the cosmic womb. By chanting this mantra, you are able to fully know yourself as SHE – mumma, lover, Shakti, pure feminine energy.

Vishwa means 'universal', *Shakti* means 'energy of Divine Mother, everything feminine in the universe (mother, daughter, lover, friend), and *Avaham* means 'come here, manifest, make it to be, let me know you are here'. *Vishwa Shakti Avaham* will call in the energy of the Divine Mumma, awakening the SHE within you.

To charge the mantra with SHE power, use your mala beads while fixing your eyes on the Sri Yantra of the Divine Mother, a sacred wheel – you can download one as part of the Lady Landscaping tools at loveyourladylandscape.com. When we work with this mantra and the Sri Yantra, we can move into the cosmic womb, so that we are inside looking out – it's pretty powerful work.

If you want to take the healing deeper, take a picture of your mumma or visualize her in your mind's eye. Each day for 21 days, say the mantra, look into her eyes, bring your hands into prayer and thank her for giving birth to you. Say, 'I forgive you, please forgive me. I love you.'

This is BIG work, especially if you've experienced a traumatic or less than positive relationship with your mumma. Each day different issues may come up, different feelings and emotions. Be with them all. Don't judge them; witness them, feel them and heal them.

~

Feel the feelings

The work, and it *is* work, is to be willing to feel ALL the feelings.

Most of us, at an early age, have learned that pain is not OK, so we've done everything we can to distance ourselves from it. We had no way of knowing how to manage the big, painful feelings of life like loneliness, heartbreak and grief so we learned really great ways not to feel them. Yes, they were mostly addictive and controlling ways, but they worked and pain was averted. Hurrah.

Except, for any kind of real healing to happen – for you, for me and for Mumma Earth – we *need* to feel them. We need to allow the painful feelings to be felt because they all have lots of important information for us. Your feelings – so many of which are stored in your womb space – are a source of inner guidance, and it's your mission should you choose to accept it, and I really recommend that you do, to get present and mindful inside your body, to be aware of what you feel, take responsibility for it and let the healing commence.

Y'see, Eve's banishment from the Garden of Eden – whatever your religion or spiritual belief – has left ladykind with a sense of universal rejection and abandonment –which is why so many of us use self-abandonment as our go-to method of protection.

When the feels get too feely, to protect ourselves from the pain, more often than not, we'll use some form of controlling behaviour. My controlling behaviour of choice was (and sometimes still is) binge eating, but the ways in which we abandon ourselves come in many, many forms:

- We stay in our heads rather than our bodies, because when we're in our heads we don't have to feel our feelings.

- We judge, shame or criticize ourselves to cover what we're feeling.

- We turn to various addictions – substance addiction, habits and behaviours to numb out.

- We hand our feelings over to someone else because we don't want to deal with them or don't know how to do so.

When we abandon ourselves in any of these ways, the wounded feelings like guilt, shame and blame, self-talk and false beliefs cause anxiety, loneliness and depression. This helps us to avoid the core feelings that we simply don't know how to, or want to handle, because… well, they're bloody painful.

The fear of feeling

Pain is not fun. Pain is not enjoyable. This is a given, right? We fear that the pain will go on for ever and that we won't be able to handle it, or we worry that if we 'go there' we'll go crazy or won't be able to function. The truth is, the only pain that goes on and on for ever is the pain we cause by how we treat ourselves.

If you're able to explore old pain or trauma – the female wound, your mumma story, your own life experiences that may have caused you pain – with BIG compassion and a deep desire to learn, connect with SHE and to bring that love and medicine IN, surprisingly, that pain can move through you really quickly.

Get curious and be loving

So let me be clear, as I said at the beginning of the book, the only intention you have to ever really set is to simply be curious: to be open to receive medicine from any situation/person/experience. And then, be willing to approach the feeling and most importantly, yourself with love. BIG LOVE.

~ Womb talk ~

Yep, this involves having an *actual* conversation with your womb. I usually take myself for a walk in the park and woodlands behind my garden, but you can do it sitting on a meditation mat or lying in bed before you get up, or in the bath. Personally, I am more open to receive when I feel held by Mumma Nature.

1. Get present in your body, take deep womb breaths (see page xxxii) and set your intention to get curious about your lady landscape. Then bring your attention to your womb space your barometer and wisdom keeper, and ask, 'What's up?'

2. Talk to her with compassion – it doesn't mean you have to use the yoga teacher voice (*aggghhhh, yoga teacher voice is the worst!*) – but imagine you have an upset child in front of you and use THAT voice to say, 'Hey love, how am I treating you?'

3. Listen for her response. She might say something like, 'I don't like that you keep saying no to things. It makes me feel lonely and unloved.'

4. Then ask SHE, 'Why are we doing that? Why do we keep saying no when we want to say hell yes?'

5. Then listen. This won't be your mind talking, so be open to what comes through. She might say, 'You think you're not good enough. You only say yes when you're good enough and you never believe you're good enough, so you never say yes.' In this scenario, you'd explore what you're avoiding feeling when you tell yourself that. Telling yourself you're not good enough for example, gives you a sense of control. If you're not good enough, you can figure out how to be better and then you can have a sense of control over things, which is, of course, an illusion – you don't have control. Not ever.

6. So, check in with your womb and then check in with SHE and ask 'What action of love can I take to feel safe?' And this is the important bit. You need to take loving action, otherwise it won't translate to your core, to your womb, to your root. When we move towards what scares us, when we're most vulnerable, we move towards our true self and that's grounded and powerful.

7. SHE might say, 'Go ring the person back and say yes.' Or perhaps, 'Dig deeper and see where you can start to loosen your grip on life – where are you holding on too tightly? What can you start without being ready?'

8. And then do the freakin' work with curiosity and love. Show yourself that you're showing up for her because that's what this is ALL about.

When you keep showing up for yourself, you develop trust and safety. Tell yourself, 'I'm not going to leave you. I'm not going to turn to food/drugs/shopping or ignore you, I'm here for you,

I'm here.' This act of self-love alone has magic powers and I've done it a lot since my mumma died. It reminds me that I have to be the one that looks out for me, stands up for me and who nurtures and supports me.

I'd suggest making this a daily practice, so that you can begin to be mindful and present in your body, then throughout the day if and when you feel a twinge of anxiety or tension, you can instantly tune in and you can ask the questions, check in with SHE and attend to it right away. Of course, this takes a lot of practice, but over time, it can becomes a strong and powerful part of your self-care practice.

~

Drop the mask, be vulnerable

When you're in your SHE power, you're less likely to feel like you need to wear that protective mask we spoke about earlier. You're more rooted in truth and so you're able to make better decisions. THIS is how we learn to love ourselves – we put our truth out there and we realize that nothing really bad happens. We then start to truly value it, instead of judging it.

When you live like this be prepared to piss people off. Not everyone is ready for a woman living her truth and expressing herself fully. It's a concept for most people, *not* a reality. There will be lots of open mouths when you call someone up and say, 'So when I said 'yes' yesterday, what I really meant was no – thank you so much for your offer though' – and don't feel the need to apologize or give a reason why. Or when you declare that you're on day 26 of your menstrual cycle, you're really gnarly and unless the person on the receiving end of your call/conversation/

email wants a no-bullshit, unfiltered response they might want to consider waiting until day 2 of your bleed. Others may make huge assumptions about you and your personality. Let them. Because you will be creating firm boundaries for yourself that feel clean and strong and straight from your root.

My practice – and it's definitely a practice that I don't always get right – is to be a true expression of how I am in any given moment – it's so powerful and it takes far less energy than trying to present a 'likeable' version of myself that's validated as 'nice' by others.

This is made much easier thanks to my connection with SHE. I used to feel very, very alone in the world before we hooked up, but now I don't have to decide things on my own. I get to trust my womb wisdom and it guides my life. SHE's pretty badass like that.

Trust yourself

We're taught to push past the wisdom of the body and ignore how it feels – it's how we've survived and strived in a dude-dominated culture. Endurance, achievement, building things, acquiring things are all rewarded, while feel-it-in-your-body-ment, which is what I call the practice of checking in with how we're physically feeling in the moment, is not.

But when you feel with ALL your senses – a super-sacred teaching from the mystery school of Isis and Magdalene – when you allow your heart, your gut and deep into your womb to be aroused, seduced, engaged, enraged, when you feel like whatever it is that you're feeling is coming from a place deeper than you, that's a physical sensation in your body that you can trust as truth – YOUR truth.

We place so many of our decisions in a thought system outside ourselves – and there are times when that's necessary – but when you focus on how it feels, you worry less about what you *should* be doing and you are led into behaviours that are coming from a more authentic place instead.

You're led by your inner knowing.
Your gut. Your fire.

This is a practice. I repeat, this is a practice.

Burn, baby, burn

In dropping the mask and learning to speak our truth, burning all the illusions and stories we've been telling ourselves can be a powerful way to set us on the path of truth and healing. Fire holds magical properties and it can be hypnotic to build a relationship with it, to feel it's majestic qualities licking at the wood and giving off heat on our face.

Fire is light and heat. It can comfort and threaten us, destroy and transform. Fire has been at the centre of ceremonies, rituals, initiations and celebrations for thousands of years, in every tribe, every civilization. But what if you could change a universal law and make fire harmless – what does that say about reality and your role in its creation? What are your limitations, really? What other possibilities remain untapped, unrealized?

The Viking and I use fire in all of our initiation ceremonies and rituals, but my favourite way to experience the power of fire is to walk on it – walking barefoot across a bed of burning coals without getting burned. Not in an Anthony Robbins 'cool moss' mind-trick way but in a powerful, intentional, overcoming fear, transformative way.

Fire walking is a powerful tool designed to help transform fear and to inspire people to do things they initially didn't think were possible. It can show you that there is more to 'reality' than you think, that many of the limitations we experience are self-imposed, and that we can create our own reality in work, in relationships and in life.

It's by far the most emotional and powerful process I know and from the moment I first set foot on hot coals in Glastonbury, UK, my life changed significantly for ever. The lighting of the fire was a ceremony – a chance to write my focus and intent on pieces of paper and place them into the flames – 'Why am I here? Who am I? Who am I to become? Then to watch as all those illusions burned through the course of the evening.

There were over 30 fire walkers the first time I walked. They all had different reasons for walking – some were doing it for charity while others were doing it to face fears, for a spiritual purpose, or in my case, to burn it all down – the fears, the limiting beliefs – and create a new beginning.

The Drummers of Avalon drummed the strong and primal beat of Mumma Earth throughout the ceremony, while our facilitator taught us how to embrace fear and make friends with it. Our aim? To create a high state of energy that would match the energy of the fire, much in the same way as the Kung Shamans who walked on fire for the empowerment and healing of their whole community.

The walk itself evoked emotion way beyond anything I'd ever expected to feel. Staring into the flames, feeling the crunch of hot coals beneath my bare feet flicked an emotional switch in me that I had set to 'off' for a while and once the tears began to flow, they didn't stop. I let go of everything as I crossed the coals. My pain, my mumma's pain, my nanna's pain. I let go of all the pain of women who have ever burned with shame or were burned alive for what they did or who they were and I let the heat of the coals and the flames of the fire cleanse me.

For 90 minutes, I sobbed. I hugged my beautiful friends who had come to cheer me on, and I sobbed. I hugged my new fire-walking buddies and I sobbed, I sat round the fire after the event listening to everyone's stories and I sobbed.

Even now, when the Viking and I do our own fire-walking events, I think about the energy raised, the emotions shared, the fears that I let go the first time I fire walked and I give thanks to the flames.

It's an honour to teach and share the sacred art of fire walking, to witness the change in the walkers as they pass through the fire. It's thrilling to be a part of the magic that unfolds. As they pass over the red-hot coals burning at over 650°C you see the old conditioning and limiting beliefs burning off, leaving underneath the true qualities of the self – confident, pure and powerful. It's total alchemy.

Don't fear the fire. BE THE FIRE.

∼ LET IT BURN ∼

You don't have to walk on fire to experience its healing, cleansing and transformative qualities, but you might want to create your own at-home burning ritual, shamana style.

Like every good witch, I have a cauldron for every occasion but a large flameproof pot, bowl or pan or outdoor fireplace will do. (Don't use one of your best saucepans though, go to a charity (thrift) store and find a big old casserole dish or stew pot that you can appropriate for ceremony.

1. Find a space outside to do your ritual – your garden or perhaps a beach – and under the dark moon, think of all the roles you take on as a woman and write them down: wife, mother, lover, writer, carer, supporter, friend, sister, auntie. Keep listing them until you run out of space.

2. Then list all the names you've ever been called that shame you, make you feel small or diminished: aggressive, fat, crazy, too much, full of yourself (*who else should you be full of – but I digress*), dramatic, not good enough, selfish, uncaring, wild, emotional, direct, too confident, bitchy, bossy, bubbly, sexy, ugly, scary... (*Just a few of what I've been called while writing this book – I'm committing them all to the flames, baby!*)

3. Sit in front of your pot or burning space, hold the paper in your hands and say each name aloud while feeling it in your body. If you're standing you could stomp Mumma Earth as you say each one.

4. When you're ready, commit it to the flames with the words, 'I release you. I am whole. I am complete. I rock.'

5. Feel the flames eating up and alchemizing that old energy into space and possibility. Let it all go. That's why you need to do this ritual outside, so the old energy can be diffused in the wind and you can feel it leaving. Doing it in a house, even with the window open, may mean that some of the energy gets stuck in a corner or behind a bookshelf, and we want it ALL to go!

6. Allow the ritual to give you a sense of completion, but make sure you honour any emotions that come up for you, too. This is powerful work. Let the pot/cauldron cool down before storing it away and make sure you nourish and ground yourself.

Best way to ground yourself after a ritual?

Sex or chocolate. Or both.

You can use this same ritual for anything specific you'd like to let go of – limiting beliefs, thoughts and feelings that are keeping you stuck. Write them down, say them out loud to SHE, the Universe, the Great Mumma, under a dark moon and then burn them into ashes.

~

Reclaiming your SHE power

Living from your fierce and feminine SHE power begins by reclaiming what's rightfully yours. If your perception of power is negative and you conjure up images of bullies and ego-driven moneymakers in slick suits, get reacquainted with what it means to be a powerful force of female good.

- **Gloria Steinem**: A writer, lecturer, political activist, feminist organizer and a frequent spokeswoman on issues of equality.

- **Kiran Gandhi**: Trained for a year in preparation for her first marathon but as race day approached, she realized she was going to be on her period on the day of the 26.2-mile run in London. She almost backed out of the marathon, but then decided to run – free-bleeding (without wearing any menstrual products like tampons or pads) the whole way through and finishing in 4:49:11 – bloody brilliant.

- **Malala Yousafzai:** Born in Pakistan and, despite receiving numerous death threats for doing so, she was an outspoken supporter of the rights of girls to have an education. In 2012 Malala was travelling home from school when the Taliban shot her in the head. Thankfully she survived, and is now a policy changer, a global advocate for female education and a Nobel Peace Prize winner.

I have NO doubt these female forces felt nervous and scared at times, they wouldn't be human if they didn't. But they trusted themselves and used their power to create lasting change. You don't have to change political policy or run a marathon without menstrual prods, but calling your power back will help you to feel more whole and complete.

~ CALL BACK YOUR SHE POWER ~

As you know, I love a ceremony so I invite you to make this as sacred as feels good to you.

First find a place that feels special to you – a forest, the sea, in front of your altar. Wear an outfit that makes you feel fierce and anoint your power points – third eye, heart, ovaries and womb space – with an essential oil blend (my SHE power scent is frankincense and rose). Finally find a talisman to represent your SHE power that you can blow your intention into – I have an amazing Allie Pohl pelvic power pendant with a lightning strike through the womb.

1. Light a candle (you can anoint it with frankincense oil for strength or rose oil for love and support) and then light it anytime you need to remind yourself of your power).

2. Take in some big, deep breaths, burn sage or Palo Santo to cleanse your auric space of any negative juju, and call in SHE, the Great Mumma, ancestors and guides to witness this calling in of your SHE power.

3. Breathe deep into your womb space through your nose and then purse your lips like you're about to whistle and release the breath fast and forcefully. With each out breath, blow out any situation/belief/person that you've allowed to stop you from claiming your power up until this moment. Take as many breaths as you need to in order to list them all and then return to a normal meditative deep breath in and out.

4. Stand barefoot (if you can) open your toes wide and root down into Mumma Earth. Bend at the knees slightly, close your eyes, have your arms to your side and your palms open to receive.

5. Now say, 'I call all of my SHE power back to me now. (Take a deep breath in and on the exhale, bring your hands into yoni mudra – the tips of both thumbs and first fingers touching and palms facing towards the body – on your womb space.)

6. 'I am whole. I am worthy. I am complete and I rock.' (Inhale and then on the exhale, bend your knees, stick your tongue out Kali Ma style and bringing hands into 'rock star' mudra – holding your middle and third finger with your thumb while the first and little fingers remain straight – RARRR!)

7. Repeat three times – or as many times as you want.

Feel free to write your own poem, chant or incantation, too – make it fierce and intentional. Things will continue to try and make you feel less than whole and powerful, so use this ritual as often as you need to.

I call my SHE power back each and every time I bleed, but you could do it every full moon to charge it with extra lunar love or on each birthday as a way to mark another trip round the sun. Keep calling your SHE power back from anywhere that its got stuck or is being held by another.

The more you do this ritual, the more situations and opportunities to express your SHE power in healthy ways will begin to show up in your world.

~

Take a dance break

Lady, you've done a LOT of work so far and when you meet yourself right where you're at, I urge you to take regular dance breaks.

A dance break is a dance-your-arse-off time-out from whatever it is that you're doing. It's good and it's necessary.

My friend Jess Grippo of jessgrippo.com is a dancer, teacher and tutu-wearing, New York-based creative badass who shares daily dance breaks via Periscope. I love receiving an alert on my phone saying, 'Jess Grippo Live: Dance Break' so that I can drop whatever it is I'm doing and shake it out with her.

Jess has a practice called the *Dance Shuffle Solution* which I love to do when I'm feeling stuck in the trying-to-figure-it-all-out-ness. I've asked her to share this simple yet powerful technique with you, too.

MUFF MUSE - JESS GRIPPO

Have you ever said the phrase, 'I'll figure it out', to yourself?

I'm retiring that phrase from my vocabulary and I encourage you to, as well.

'Figuring it out' implies a heady maths equation, a mental exercise in sorting out the puzzle pieces and thinking of the best way to arrange them. This is a great tactic when it comes to actual equations or puzzles, but it's a terrible approach to real life situations.

Real life requires ALL of us – not just our heads. When you lose your job, when you are going through a break-up or a health challenge, when you wake up feeling 'blah' day after day... this is the stuff of life that can't be 'figured out'.

The alternate approach I've discovered is to literally and figuratively 'dance into the answers'. To dance requires utilizing your whole body, channelling your emotions and moving your soul. It quiets the chattering mind and opens you up to spaciousness, new possibilities and rhythm, i.e. answers that you would've never discovered had you stayed stiff and in your head.

At the simplest level, you can stop what you're doing in any moment, put on some music and just dance. My favourite exercise for this is what I call the 'Dance Shuffle Solution' and here's how it goes:

1. *Start by getting in touch with the question or dilemma you are facing.*

2. *Hit SHUFFLE on your iPod or online playlist.*

3. *Commit to dancing to whatever the next three songs are that come up. The point is for you not to know what songs are going to come next, so that you just let your body respond to the music.*

Afterwards, it's great to do some free writing or just sit in silence and integrate what happened in your dance. Sometimes answers come in the form of a new idea, sometimes through the lyrics in one of the songs, sometimes through a new desire or impulse that moves through you.

Try it out!

Treat life as a dance and waltz your way into answers you never even imagined! It's quite a magical process.

LADY LANDSCAPING TOOLS

SHE medicine

- **Connect with your womb space.** Get in touch with your SHE power daily through breath, touch and conversation – this will help you to create a lifelong relationship with her.

- **Hear The Call.** Become a Called Girl – someone who, despite the endless stream of information you receive each day, is able to cultivate her SHE power and trust her own rooted wisdom as truth.

- **Let yourself feel it to heal it.** You know that patriarchy has caused some big wounds, but when you begin the work of healing yourself, you heal all those who have gone before and all of those who are yet to come.

Mantra

Repeat this mantra any time you need a reminder:

'The safest place to be is in my body.'

**#*bloodyconversationstarters*

These can be used as journal prompts, dive deeper questions, book club or SHE circle themes or, y'know actual bloody conversation starters on social media, with:

- What is *your* relationship with your lady parts?

- What would happen if you dropped your mask – the game face you wear for the world – and allow yourself to be seen and vulnerable?

- What does the term SHE power mean to you?

Read

Tsultrim Allione, *Feeding Your Demons*

Louise Hay, *The Power Is Within You*

C.J. Johnson, *Wombology*

Monica Sjoo and Barbara, Mor, *The Great Cosmic Mother*

Marianne Williamson, *A Woman's Worth*

PART II

KNOW YOUR LADY LANDSCAPE

The REDvolution
starts here!

CHAPTER 4

SHE Cycles

*'The wild nature carries the bundles for healing; she
carries everything a woman needs to be and know.
She carries the medicine for all things. She carries
stories and dreams and words and songs and signs
and symbols. She is both vehicle and destination.'*

CLARISSA PINKOLA ESTES

I heart Mumma Nature. She is a force of cyclic power, which reminds me over and over again that I am her and SHE is me.

The seasons, the cycles of life and death, moon cycles – we are ruled by her cycles and women have a menstrual cycle, our very own incredible internal map that can give us direction and guidance on everything we do.

For thousands of years, a woman's menstrual cycle was part of the natural rhythm of life. We were our own timekeepers with our very own information services, but sadly, we've lost connection to our cyclic nature.

Our roots have been pulled from Mumma Nature – we eat fruit out of season, we plan our rest time in the form of a one or two-week holiday and weekend getaways – we've abandoned our cycles and replaced them with control and sameness.

We've let society create our reality by plugging into phones and technology that tell us we need to do, act and feel the same and that we should buy things to make ourselves 'feel better'.

I'm not saying we should all wear tie-dye and Birkenstocks and burn patchouli incense, but since our roots have been disconnected from Mumma Earth, a deep disconnect from ourselves has been created and it's shown up as painful and uncomfortable menstrual cycles, shame about being a woman, gnarly PMT and reproductive issues.

We're no longer letting our cyclic nature guide us, we're letting the pain and dis-ease we suffer each month control us, and we're determined to prove that if we can just do it all – mummahood, career, relationships – we'll be worthy of admiration, adoration and respect.

The thing is, you ARE worthy of admiration, adoration and respect RIGHT NOW simply by being a woman. It's just that we live in a solar based, masculine society – one where the emphasis is to strive and do and be successful, and this isn't a place that's truly comfy for us, at least not all the time.

Women are cyclical.
Women are flow.
Women are fluid.

Women are not consistent. (For so long we've been told that this is a sign of weakness, when really it's a super power, it means at each phase of our menstrual cycle, we show up to life differently and a whole set of different skills and abilities become available to us in each of those phases.)

We are not linear. We are not meant to 'do' ALL the time. As we move through the different phases of our menstrual cycle

– managed by different hormones – we move through different energy levels, moods and needs.

The first half of your menstrual cycle, the follicular phase, is masculine. This is typically a time for big energy, amped-up creativity and when you're much more able to think in straight lines. The second half of your cycle, the luteal phase, is feminine, a time when you begin to move inwards and want to withdraw from the world. You crave quiet and feel a deep need for contemplation.

Unfortunately, very few of us even know this about ourselves or, if we do, we believe that we will be less productive, less useful, if we allow ourselves to follow the rhythm of our menstrual cycle – our inner guidance system. Instead we try our best to do it like a dude, we try to maintain the masculine, go-for-it energy throughout the entire cycle, but by doing so, we're are ignoring our fundamental needs as women and we barely survive the second half of our cycle.

Feel the fear

Our bodies, if we let them, are deeply in tune with the cycles of the seasons, the elements and the moon.

By not rolling with our natural rhythms, more women than ever are feeling subtle, yet persistent anxiety, depression or exhaustion, they're suffering from stress, burnout and more alarmingly, menstrual related health problems. We're cultivating a dude-like existence – creating things we can control, striving hard, doing things in a linear way – and this results in us losing touch with our SHE power. And our SHE power is the power to see and embrace things that are beyond our control, the things that our heart and womb yearns for – intimacy, creative expression, authenticity, sisterhood and meaningful contribution. It's no wonder that we suffer so much stress in modern life; our energies – physical, mental, emotional and creative – have been forced into a structure that doesn't go with our feminine flow.

And I get it. There's fear.

Fear that it's not in the interest of a patriarchal and consumer-led society to 'let' women realize and own their SHE power.

Fear of what might be unleashed if every woman were to wake up to her innate SHE power, grow roots and rise.

It's why – understandably so – few women dare to go there. The imprints of being burned at the stake, being stoned, our truths untold and our stories edited and silenced, have been etched on our ovaries and we're scared.

For a long time, I explored the edges of who I was as a woman, in this body, at this time in my work. I scratched the surface, I tried things out, I shared some stories online about menstruation, but I always erred on the side of caution. Not wanting to offend, say the wrong thing or risk someone not liking me. When SHE called, I was all, 'What? You want me to really go there? As in ovary-deep, mud wrestling go there? No thanks, I rather like my comfy online world of body-love and self-esteem.'

Well, you can see how THAT turned out.

Go there. SHE has your back.

The lady code

Every day since I released *Code Red*, the go-to guide for understanding and unlocking your monthly super powers, I have received mail and messages from women around the world thanking me for sharing my work about the menstrual cycle but also expressing their deep, deep anger.

'Why was I not told this as a girl?' 'Why is this not taught in schools?' 'Why have I being denied my super powers?'

I hear you, sisters.

In a world where we're constantly being sold new and ridiculous ways to improve ourselves and make ourselves better, you have a unique-to-you lady code that once unlocked, will give you access to everything you need to create a bloody amazing life except until now, patriarchy has kept the key in a box with the lid closed tight shut.

This isn't a new concept or another modern health trend but an ancient wisdom, passed down through our blood, and every time we bleed we have access to its power.

Basically this shiz is sacred and my job as your guide-ess and menstrual maven is to make this wisdom totally accessible and most importantly, relevant to us as modern women.

Most of us are tired of constantly pushing against our natural rhythms, we've lost our connection to our SHE power – our vital creative life force – and we've been seduced into thinking that PMT, pain, or any other lady-part dis-ease is 'normal', something we have to endure, something that comes with the territory of being a woman.

Yet, there's a whole unexplored part of our lady landscape and our entire experience of being a woman is out of whack because we're working against it and that's causing emotional and physical trauma in our bodies.

We ALL bleed.

It's the red thread that connects us.

It's sacred.

It's messy.

It's powerful.

**Hey Patriarchy, call us Pandora,
we've got the key to our box
and we're going to open it.**

The cycles of woman

To fully understand our menstrual cycle we need to first understand the cycles of being a woman.

Dream on, dreamer

You move from girl to woman at menarche (your first bleed) and this signals the opening of your second chakra, *svadhistana*, in your pelvic area (for more about the chakras see page 180). High fives, your spiritual life force, kundalini, has awoken. You're a woman now and the menstrual cycle – which you'll experience roughly 450 cycles between now and menopause – will, if you let it, unfold teachings each and every cycle. It's a jumble of growth and learning, and the space where dreams and ambition are first created. Feelings of Wonder Woman-like invincibility are strong and you are frequently told that the 'world is your oyster'. Whatever that actually means.

Manifesting maven

Next you enter what's known as your 'fertile' years, this is when you become the creatrix, mistress of your destiny. You can birth, grow, create and nurture *anything* into being – children, a career, art, a home, ANYTHING. You navigate life and its challenges and you are in a cycle of perpetual learning, growing, manifesting and letting go.

The transformational years

After you have played out the parts society dictates you fulfil – a brief career stint followed by motherhood – your requirement is then, again by society, rendered redundant. You are no more. At a time in your life when you are evolving emotionally and psychologically, you are rejected physically.

Ah, the transformational, perimenopause years.

Fuck society. This should be the most powerful phase in the cycle of woman, it's when you have learned all the lessons from your cyclical unfolding and are ready to own your throne as the wise, wild and fully expressed woman that you are. This phase represents a time of shedding old conditioned ideas of who you *should* be and instead really becoming an expression of your true self.

It's not easy to age in our society, in fact it's positively discouraged and frowned on. It's why so many women suffer during this phase, because we're told to fear getting older, to fight age with surgery and cosmetics, to deny the story that is playing out in our wrinkles. But if you attempt to halt the physical aging process, there's a good chance you'll be ridiculed for your efforts or called names, if you dare to express yourself in a way that isn't deemed 'age appropriate' by the media.

The wise woman

Your wise years, your post-menopausal phase, is when you fully own your power – you no longer have to do the inner work. Some of my most favourite teachers are post-menopausal women. You are unedited, unfiltered and share deep no-bullshit knowing, which is the only kind of teaching we ever really need. Yet so many of our elders and wise women are ignored or disrespected by society.

They feel invisible to a world that's obsessed by looks and youth, when they should be revered for all that they are, know and share.

Now, we spend roughly between 25–30 years experiencing the energy of these cycles of woman through our own monthly menstrual cycle. Yep, every month we experience the opportunity to dream and plant new seeds, to manifest and create, to transform and let go, and to share wisdom, so when we are made to feel redundant after menopause it's easy to see to why so many of us are also suffering in the pre-menstrual and menstrual phases of our cycle.

Our own cycle is a reflection of what's happening in the wider lady landscape.

The RED-volution starts here

Until very recently, menstruation was perceived as taboo and – despite working with women who are embracing their cycle and learning to love their lady landscapes – I'm reminded on a near daily basis that talking about periods in what my mumma used to call my 'outside voice', is still pretty freakin' radical.

The good news? The RED-volution is ON!

Women are beginning to talk openly about their periods on social media, books like *Code Red* are selling thousands of copies and are featured in mainstream media and magazines like *Nylon* and *Rookie* talk about menstruation as a 'sacred act'. New feminism is coming round to the idea that we don't have to be the 'same' as, or 'equal' to, dudes, understanding that our true power is in being cyclic, and not being hard on ourselves when we're unable to deliver in the same linear, goal-centric way that dudes do. (*Of course, we CAN deliver like that, but only for a finite amount of time* until we break/suffer pain and discomfort and that serves no one, least of all you.)

Lena Dunham speaks openly about periods, endometriosis and uteruses. As I mentioned earlier, Kiran Gandhi, the drummer from MIA, ran the London marathon free bleeding (see page 66) – so making 'free bleeding' an actual thing. I work with clients who dare to have the bloody conversations and the #sharemycycle hashtag is an opportunity for women to share what day they're on in their menstrual cycle and it's used globally to discuss the menstrual experience online. TV shows, plays and zines are talking about bleeding, too; these would previously have been seen as fringe, but are now being received in the mainstream. It's a positive start, but it's going to take all of us having the bloody conversations and using our 'outside voices' – loudly and often – to bring about a real and lasting change.

So let's bloody do it, yeah? Let's surf the crimson wave.

The bloody basics

Each month, meaning each menstrual month, the time between each bleed can become a map for charting the optimal times for everything from going on a date, writing copy for your website, having an awkward conversation with your partner to having great sex, asking for a raise or taking a nap.

SHE TRUTH

Your menstrual cycle isn't just the days that you bleed, it's the entire menstrual month, and it makes total sense that you get to know it and then use it to optimize your awesome-ness.

Your menstrual cycle can be mapped in the same way as the cycles of the moon and the seasons. When you begin to see your monthly cycle as a SHE power activator and not something you have to endure, you become a cyclic sister who has monthly super powers that can create a bloody amazing life. (*Wearing a Lycra costume, cracking a lasso and calling yourself Wonder Woman is totally optional.*)

The menstrual cycle governs the feminine flow, not only of each monthly bleed, but also of information, emotions, spirituality and creativity. It shows us that in each phase, we have access to incredible super powers that can be used to enhance our lives and express ourselves more fully. When we notice these changing energies and adjust our lives to live in harmony with them, we have an amazing opportunity to be creative and achieve success (whatever that looks like for you) in a far more SHE-led way.

For example, this is the second book I've written in complete sync with the powers of my cycle. I know that during my premenstrual phase, I get *really* truthful so my writing becomes much more from the womb and the words flow much easier, I have a creative cosmic nudge that I don't experience so loudly, if at all, during other phases. It doesn't mean that I can't write during the other phases of my cycle, it just means that I have a monthly super power that I use to help me write with ease.

Getting to know your cycle is crucial to your health, work, relationships and overall wellbeing. The ebb and flow of our dreams, creativity and hormones in each phase of our cycle offer us a profound opportunity to deepen our connection with our inner knowledge and to live in balance with the different creative energies that occur each month. What would life be like if you knew that you could use your pre-ovulation phase to plan your workload for the month and that in ovulation you are queen of communication? How about knowing you can use the pre-menstrual phase to get to the heart of what works and what doesn't and during menstruation, assess and review? Cool, huh?

This is just the beginning, if you want to know everything that each phase has to offer, you're going to need to chart. Charting isn't just the territory of those who want to get pregnant; your cycle is a gold mine of incredible insight that will provide information on how best to use your energy, your intuition and your SHE power. (Download a printable cycle chart with instructions on how to fill it in and use it at: loveyourladylandscape.com). I've been charting for a long time now, and with each monthly menstrual cycle, I learn a little bit more about myself as a woman in the world. The more I learn, the more I'm able to fully claim my powers, care for myself, articulate my experience and live my life in ways that feel good and meaningful.

Knowing that something SHE-led and divine is unfolding in me has made me far more accepting of my tendencies, my body and myself. My relationship with my bleed cycle has quite literally, brought me home.

When you work with your menstrual cycle and unlock this wisdom and the medicine that is within it, you are setting out on a sacred journey deep into yourself, one that ladykind has been travelling since the beginning of time.

Many of us are told that our menstrual cycle is the 5–7-day period of bleeding and it's this bleed time that's become known as our 'time of the month', but lady, 'your time' is ALL freaking month. In fact, virtually every part of your body is affected during every stage of your menstrual cycle – pulse rate, blood pressure, body temperature, even the frequency of how often you need to pee – are effected by it 365 days a year.

Now, just like the moon, your menstrual cycle follows roughly a 29-day cycle and in the same way that the moon waxes, and wanes, so do we.

Each month, we take a journey through both the light and the dark parts of ourselves; we get the chance to renew and refresh our entire being – physically, mentally, psychologically and spirituality.

In fact, in many indigenous tribes, the word for 'moon' and 'menstruation' are interchangeable and that's because most societies have, at one time or another, understood the link between women's menstrual cycles and the moon. This book and the practices in it is your invitation to remember that you, too, know this to be true.

The moon cycle

As women in the world, we're ruled by the moon – she is the primary symbol for female energy – so it makes total sense for us to chart *La Luna's* cycle, what with her taking about 29 days to circle the Earth, the same amount of time as the average woman's menstrual cycle.

Waxing moon

When the moon is 'waxing', it's getting larger in the sky, moving from the new moon towards the full moon. This is the time to start new projects, meet new people, conceptualize ideas and attract new love. The waxing moon phase lasts about 14 days.

Full moon

When the moon is full, she forms a perfect silvery sphere of gorgeousness in the sky. This is a time for 'getting it on' – you'll feel super-frisky, but just know, your fertility will be heightened too. Be prepared! It's also a powerful time to manifest and bring dreams into being. The period of the full moon lasts from about three days before, to three days after, the actual full moon.

Waning moon

The waning moon is decreasing in size, moving from the full moon towards the new moon. This is the perfect time to break bad habits or addictions, to end unhealthy relationships and to really tap deep into your intuition.

New moon/dark moon

This is when the moon is directly between the Earth and the Sun, and therefore hidden. This is a great time for planning new beginnings and new undertakings, while having a little 'cave time' to read, watch movies and pamper your sweet self.

Getting in sync with the moon

The wise women before us were in total sync with the moon, they knew that our period is highly affected by the moon's movement. Their blood and hormonal cycle followed its ebb and flow. From new moon to full moon, as the cycle waxed, oestrogen levels increased leading to super-charged fertility when the moon was at her fullest, roundest and most abundant. From full moon to new moon, the waning half of the cycle, progesterone dominated and led to the release of blood at the dark moon.

Today, we are totally out of sync with the moon's cycles. We get so busy in our daily lives that for the most part, we ignore the cyclic changes of Mumma Nature – the seasons, the moon, the ebb and flow of the tides – all of which are indicative as to how we should be living. Our menstrual cycle is often medicated with synthetic hormones and not allowed to flow naturally from our body because we stuff it with a tampon, we suppress any resulting pain and symptoms with Western medicine, which means we are ignoring the messages that Mumma Nature, our body and our cycle are giving us and when we do that? Shit will, and does, hit the fan. In other words, we get stressed out, exhausted, depleted, depressed.

We silence the deep, ancient, feminine wisdom by using caffeine, drugs, TV and social media to create destructive cycles of self-medication, cycles that keep us locked into the myth that being a woman is hard work, that it's painful and that any alternative involving resting or not striving so hard is seen as weak.

Take a look outside the window right now – what season is your part of the Earth currently experiencing? What are the characteristics of that season? Is it winter? Maybe the trees are bare and you've had to come inside for warmth and light, or perhaps it's spring and everything feels new and vital.

When we tune in to the cycles of the season, in the same way that we can map our menstrual cycle using the phases of the moon, we can use the seasons to deepen our understanding of our bleed cycle, too.

Cycle phases 101

Your menstrual cycle really *IS* the most extraordinary self-care tool, and charting it, exploring it, getting to know it, beginning to build a relationship with your needs, wants and tendencies in each part of the cycle, is vital, and not just the first two phases that we're most familiar with.

On a super-practical, day-to-day basis, it means you're able to navigate your life from a place of power but, on a spiritual and emotional level, it can crack you wide open to connecting with SHE, with your body and with your lady landscape.

So, download the SHE Flow cycle chart in the Lady Landscaping Toolkit (see page 251) on day 1 of your blood, crack open a journal, check where the moon is at and begin an ever-unfolding journey of self-discovery.

Think of yourself like Dorothy in *The Wizard of Oz* each and every month, except your path isn't yellow, it's blood red.

Oh and one last thing, if you are on the pill, or you no longer cycle due to menopause or surgically induced menopause, this doesn't mean that you miss out on the cycle action insight and wisdom. While your body won't be experiencing a menstrual bleed, it will still experience its own cycles but these may be much subtler, so to fully embrace the cyclic energy, I'd recommend working with the phases of the moon to experience the energy of each phase – I've highlighted which menstrual phase is represented by which moon phase. All the traits, archetypes and super powers are the same; it's just that through your menstrual cycle, you experience these through your body and through your blood, making the practice of cycling – no bike required – totally unique to you.

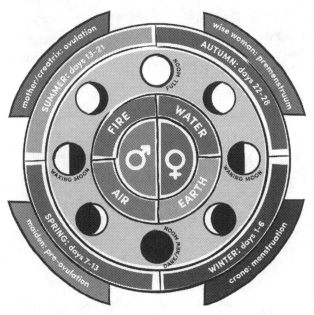

Your menstrual cycle

Pre-ovulation

- **Lunar:** Waxing moon

- **Season:** Spring

- **Archetype:** Maiden

- **Days:** 7–13

Pre-ovulation is the first phase of your cycle and usually begins around day 7 all the way through to day 13. Obviously, this will vary depending on the length of your cycle and it may take a few months of charting to really start to see where each phase begins and ends, but that's part of your very own lady landscape exploration!

You've just bled, and now there's potential to start afresh. We are SO lucky, that each month, we get the opportunity to start over. After the heaviness of our bleed, there's freshness to this time of the menstrual month — it feels positive, we're able to start planning with clearness and clarity. You will start to come out of your winter-like cocoon, the steady increase in oestrogen boosts your brain's serotonin levels, which leads to an increase in energy and enthusiasm for... well, just about everything and you'll feel a lot more upbeat than you did in your previous bleed days. Hurrah.

In fact, you'll be pretty much rockin' and rulin'. You may want to go out dancing and bust some moves, hook up with girlfriends or go on dates. Your verbal abilities heighten in this phase too, words come easily, you're articulate and can pack a witty one-liner, so if you've got a big presentation or an important call to make, definitely do it in this phase of your cycle.

Pre-ovulation super powers

- You have the memory, logic and reasoning to understand projects fully and, more importantly, you also have the drive and determination to make them happen.

- Your physical energy is very masculine, which means stamina is renewed, and you are active and engaged in life. You can rock out on the dance floor, in the gym and most definitely in the bedroom.

- Take risks — there is no better time than during pre-ovulation, your enthusiasm and lust for life in this phase makes anything seem possible.

- You are a powerhouse of creativity and you can work for longer to get shit done. If you're going to pull an all-nighter, this is the phase to do it in.

- You want to be seen and heard. You are fearless, self-confident and full of self-belief, so your energy is very upfront and high-spirited. This phase of your cycle is masculine, it's active and engaged and has a neon light above it that flashes 'watch out world, here I come.'

Ovulation

- **Lunar:** Full moon

- **Season:** Summer

- **Archetype:** Mother

- **Days:** 13–21

At ovulation, a tiny egg is released from one of your two ovaries – they alternate from one cycle to the next – making it the time you are most likely to get pregnant – you've been warned. Wink.

This is the second phase of your cycle and usually begins around day 13 all the way through to day 21, and throughout it you'll be flashing like a neon sign, 'I'm hot-to-trot, come and get me!' and that's because g-friend, you're ovulating.

Since day 1 of your cycle, oestrogen and testosterone have been doing all they could to play cupid. That upbeat, high-energy, optimistic mood they've been dishing out all through your pre-ovulation phase wasn't just a high five and 'we think you're awesome' from biology. It was a rather sneaky trick, a clever ploy, to get you to either land yourself a man or to overlook the foibles of one you may already spend time with, so you'd keep him around at least until day 13, when the possibility for pregnancy is super-high in women who don't take any form of contraception. It also happens to be when oestrogen and testosterone reach their highest peaks during your entire cycle. What this means is that the optimism, the confidence, the personal power, the extroversion, the 'doing' mentality, the fun-loving attitude that has all been growing since day 1 of your cycle is now peaking, too. Oh yeah, you're high-octane baby and basically queen o' the universe. You take things less personally, you're able to get shit done with ease, you want to socialize and it's a time in your cycle when you're happy to be seen.

Ovulation super powers

- You can be totally captivating in any situation. Think Marilyn Monroe in *The Seven Year Itch*. I know, right? Guaranteed Marilyn was ovulating when she did the scene with THAT dress and the air vent.

- You can take on the world super-woman style. (Lycra as always when I talk of superheroes, which I do a LOT, is optional.)

- You get called a lucky bitch because, well, things just naturally go your way. No drama, just awesome results.

- You have the power to conjure up your dream job, ideal clients or maybe even a cheeky hot date. In fact, whatever you really desire, there isn't a doubt that you can make it happen at this time.

Pre-menstruation

- **Lunar:** Waning moon

- **Season:** Autumn (fall)

- **Archetype:** Wise and wild woman

- **Days: 23–28** (or start of menstruation)

This is the third phase of your cycle and if your egg wasn't fertilized during ovulation, from roughly day 23 through to your bleed, you will experience a withdrawal from all three of the following hormones – oestrogen, testosterone and progesterone.

Now, decreasing oestrogen is the one that cause bouts of nervousness, anxiety, teary-ness and the blues due to the reduction in mood-stabilizing serotonin, which also spells the return of noradrenaline.

Cue boos and hisses, because this is the pantomime baddie of the hormone world. If something irritates you – like your partner spilling red wine on your new carpet – just know that your temper and your partner are about to get fully acquainted.

Meanwhile, withdrawing progesterone has you weeping at… well, just about anything. And after the high-octane levels you've been experiencing in the previous two weeks, testosterone withdrawal brings in feelings of self-doubt about your appearance and your abilities. Is it any wonder so many women hate on this part of their cycle?

The good news is that despite the cramps, the mood swings and the 'I'm-not-good-enough' on repeat loop, this phase does have super-powers – you can find love for it, and for some, including myself, it can end up being the phase of your cycle that you look forward to the most.

Honest.

Just as in nature's autumn, the light of the summer is dimming and we're called to spend more time inside. You may find yourself wanting to clean the house, or getting more annoyed than usual at a partner or a child for leaving their dirty clothes on the landing – yes, hot Viking husband, I'm talking to you.

Pre-menstruation super powers

- You can trust your intuition to guide you in making big-ass life decisions because your bullshit detector is set to maxim-o.

- Your psychic abilities are heightened. (*Yep, and you don't have to wear a headscarf and big silver hoop earrings to do it either. Unless you want to, obvz.*)

- You can make bitchcraft a positive thing because speaking your heart-truth doesn't have to rude or offensive.

- You can move through creative blocks, meet deadlines and get super-organized.

- You can spot a problem and you have the creative fire and inspiration to fix it.

- You get the opportunity to be charmed and potentially a li'l bit dangerous (when I say dangerous I'm talking the truth-telling enchantress kind) EVERY month.

- Your intuition and psychic abilities heighten making you a charmed and dangerous enchantress – a truth seeking, cut the bullshit, mistress of bitchcraft. Basically, you're hot shit.

SHE TRUTH

If these powers aren't harnessed, there's a chance they can manifest as pain, anger or perceived craziness. If you're able to work with them, lady, you become a super-charged, power source for truth.

Menstruation

- **Lunar:** Dark/new moon

- **Season:** Winter

- **Meaning:** Crone

- **Days:** 1–6 (or end of menstruation)

If you're not pregnant, you'll be bleeding. This is day 1 of your cycle, and depending on your particular cycle, your bleed can last anything for 3–8 days. During this week, oestrogen starts out at rock bottom and begins a steady climb. The first days may leave you feeling achy and tired, but from day 3 onwards, you'll experience a boost in your energy, mood, optimism and brain skills.

When oestrogen rises, it also boosts your levels of testosterone, and when this increases, it pumps up your self-assured feelings like confidence and courage – but don't get too excited, on the days of your bleed these happiness hormones, while taking the lift to the top, are still only at the first floor, so as these hormones dipped and called you into yourself during your pre-menstrual phase, the first 3 or 4 days of your bleed are calling you to rest and to immerse yourself in self-care and preservation.

Winter is the dark moon of our cycle, a time to retreat and to honour this sacred time of bleeding. I know that's really hard to do when we all live such busy lives, but acknowledging your bleed, if only for an hour, will give you such incredible insight into yourself. How we look after ourselves and be with ourselves during this time can really set the story for the rest of the cycle.

**Operating and functioning in the
outside world during your bleed
can become much more difficult.
That's because you're not meant to.**

Menstruation super powers

- You instinctively know the best direction in life to take, as you are super-clear about your purpose in life

- You are able to connect to SHE/source directly, and identify and release the stuff that no longer serves you

- You can restore your sexual, creative and spiritual energy.

- You can cope easily with change, and you're able to forgive and forget with ease. You're a witch, a sorceress, an all-powerful woman.

SHE TRUTH

Wouldn't it be worth changing deadlines and slowing down during your bleed to allow your intuitive self to provide you with insight and creative ideas, to connect with SHE to get clarity at a soul level about your purpose and to have the commitment to action it?

Honouring my menstruation phase has probably been my biggest revelation since charting and working with my cycle. I surrender to my flow. When I honour and surrender to it, I am gifted with so many signs and messages into how to move forwards with a situation, what direction to take in my life, that I no longer worry about what I should be doing or where I should be going. If I have a big-ass decision to make, I simply bleed on it. In fact, sometimes when people ask me as to whether I'd like to take up a new role or be part of a project or collaboration, I'll tell them to let me bleed on it, and I'll get back to them straight after. This is how I do business and it's how I do life. I bleed on it. I really recommend it.

Go with your flow

One of the many great things about working with your cycle is that you'll realize there's not a one-size-fits-all way of working, eating, having sex, making money, talking to your partner.

As I've said before a cyclic woman isn't linear, she's liminal and at each phase in the cycle her needs, wants, desires and energy and hormone levels are different. So for example, if you've ever taken up running and were like 'hell no, this isn't for me', it might be worth trying it again during your pre-ovulation phase when your energy levels are high and you feel able to take on new challenges. This is because in your pre-menstrual phase, your body will feel a lot less love for pounding the pavement for 5 miles and will be craving a softer, more feminine movement practice.

Don't you love how this all works?

Your menstrual cycle is your very own amazing inner teacher, guide, initiator and spiritual practice right in your womb – it's like a Filofax (*do they still exist?*) of wisdom, creativity and insight, an oracle of awesome and the most incredible self-care tool. On a super-practical, day-to-day basis it means you're able to navigate your life from a place of power, but on a spiritual and emotional level, it can crack you wide open to self-discovery. The real fun begins when you start identifying your own super powers and hot spots in each phase.

For example, I know that on Day 18, I am hot-to-trot so I will ALWAYS make sure there is space in my diary for a date with the hot Viking. On days 14 and 15 I am super articulate and productive, so I book in as many meetings and interviews and speaking gigs here. And on day 25 I am Kali Ma incarnate, I am RAGE-full so the Viking throws chocolate at me from a distance. These are just a few of the super powers and hotspots that unravelled as I began to chart. What you soon realize is that you'll never need a self-help book again, because your cycle is your very own YOU-nique-to-you treasure map.

Hint: YOU are the treasure.

Rewilding

Now, as a Scorpio, I LOVE the darkness of all things, so it makes total sense that I do this work because in esoteric medicine, the passionate and intense Scorpio rules the reproductive organs and it's in the dark, second half of your menstrual cycle where Scorpio-like tendencies can be fully expressed – mood swings, truth-telling, sharp tongue – recognize any of those?

If someone is super-perky, I will want to know why. I will want to scratch the surface and get underneath their glossy exterior because that part of me will not believe for one minute that people can actually be like that. (I'm not saying it's right by the way, either, it's just a tendency of mine.) Also, since my parents have died, I've got very little time or patience for small talk. I always want to meet people on a deeper level, so I want to see their vulnerability, their anger, their truth in ALL its forms. In fact, for a while there I spent a

LOT of time in the darkness and people were really worried about me, but I was fully aware that what I was feeling was cyclic and that, as always, the light would return at some point. And it did, because it always does.

I think our society is so susceptible to believing that practising yoga, eating kale or drinking a green juice is going to help them transcend darkness and bring them into the light, when what actually happens is that they end up getting really uptight and defensive about their path because they're fighting an inner battle to suppress their darkness.

There's no way to bypass it. It's why we have night and day, it's why the moon waxes and wanes, it's why each month you have the light and dark phase of your menstrual cycle – Mumma Nature's reminders that no one is exempt from the darkness.

What if you got into a relationship with the darkness? Faced the aspects of you that you criticize, try to fix or get rid of?

Here's where SHIT... GETS... REAL...

It's often said, mainly by my husband, that I come without a filter and do you know what? I make no apologies for that.

I honour the voice that's inside me.

If I'm angry, I won't act like I'm not.

If I disagree with something I won't condone it simply to keep the peace.

If I'm worried or nervous, I won't put on a positive face to make others feel at ease.

When I'm raging and angry, oftentimes friends or family members will try to have me watch what I say, or help me to at least moderate it or try to get me to a place where I lose the initial trigger as to what made me angry in the first place, but this just makes me MORE pissed. Because when we ignore our anger, passion and true feelings, when we don't allow them to be fully felt and expressed IN and THROUGH our body, we sell ourselves out of the FULL experience of being a woman.

We become a shell of our wholeness.

I get it.

It's risky to share and express ourselves.

It's imprinted in our ovaries to be fearful of telling our truth. Yet I bet you feel a fire deep in your womb and belly, righteous anger, the heat of NOT telling your truth, of biting your tongue, of suppressing your anger, of trying to live a life of love and light. It may even show itself as a physical manifestation – anxiety, depression, rashes or a 'down-there' dis-eases like endometriosis, PCOS or fibroids.

Y'see, telling your truth is the only thing TO do.

But we've been tamed and censored and never is it more present than in the pre-menstrual phase of our menstrual cycle, because it's here that our womanly wildness – our truth, our voice, our very essence in all it's messy and imperfect glory – demands to be untamed and uncensored.

Now, if that *really* happened, if we took life by the ovaries and spilled our heart, gut and womb out without censorship, the patriarchal societies in which most of us live would be scared shitless.

We'd be dangerous. Except we wouldn't, not really, we'd simply be in our truth.

What's more dangerous to me is that so many of us have disowned the second half of our menstrual cycle. If the first half is a deep inhale, the second half is the exhale, the let go – an opportunity to stop doing and to 'be'. To let our heart, gut and womb lead us in a different, deeper way of being, and yet so many of us are totally disconnected from it.

Why?

This phase can get messy – truth doesn't come tied in a pretty manageable bow – and as modern women we learn very early on to keep the 'messy' aspects of femininity under wraps. Our emotions, should they spill out, get squashed and we apologize. A LOT.

We worry that we're being seen as too much, while struggling with feeling not enough.

We're scared to come undone and we cling to the safe space, but there are no safe spaces.

This is why the practice of rewilding is so important. We need to restore and protect our natural processes and that involves being willing to come undone. Over and over again… When I began my own rewilding adventure I was scared. I thought I was 'too much', that I was taking up space and that I was just too fucking emotional, but slowly, with each cycle, I started to really explore the rage, the bitchiness, the uncensored nature of my very being and my pre-menstrual/waning moon phase has now become my mentor in truly owning my voice and speaking my truth.

SHE TRUTH

Not everyone will dig you for rewilding, and at first it may feel overwhelming, but we'll take it slow and drink in our wild and free nature like a fine Mary Magdalene approved red wine, 'K?

It's why our menstrual cycle, this incredible inner map, provides us with the opportunity each month to come into a place of darkness with ourselves, to allow these things that in other parts of the cycle we'd be afraid to see, to show up.

Most of us have grown up totally detached from our intuition, our innate feminine wisdom and intelligence system, so we can easily override this pre-menstrual phase. If you take the pill you'll know that you can shut off from your cycle completely, which means you effectively silence your entire inner GPS system so that you can exist fully in the solar part of your cycle.

The wisdom of our body, our intuition, the feminine aspects of our very existence are denied and judged as second rate because we live in a world that demands scientific proof for everything – to back up our own experience of what it is to be a woman. We write off the possibility that our direct experience is valid, that our intuition and knowledge is relevant, yet we need both.

We are afraid to see the truth, what it might mean to have to admit a shortcoming or make a change in our life, people HATE change, yet this pre-menstrual phase is Kali Ma incarnate, and she demands change.

I am woman, hear me roar

The wild and wise woman archetype is your guide-ess through rewilding. She invites you to explore your natural instincts as a woman – your innate deep knowing and universal wisdom. When you go against your cyclic, authentic nature your suffering is inevitable. You may be so far removed from your natural knowing that it can take years of unravelling pain, hurt and wounds before you finally hear her call and go home to your wild woman self to heal. She is always calling for us, welcoming us back to the place we know as truth, our core wilderness.

What is your instant response to rewilding? How does the wild and wise woman archetype manifest in you? Do you suppress her? Does she feel so uncontrollable you have to keep her on a leash?

Have you even met her yet? I invite you to get still with yourself, take in some big beautiful breaths and allow yourself to meet her.

Your cycle is a conduit.

If we let it, our womb and menstrual cycle will constantly feed us messages and information that we need in order to navigate our lives skilfully. But instead of allowing ourselves to be guided by this, we often allow the thoughts that run through our heads, run the entire show that is our life. We don't allow our emotions and bodily sensations to be fully felt and processed and then act accordingly. It's why so many of us are quick to judge, because we're reacting from thoughts, not responding from our own pussy-led truth.

We work from the top down, and not from the womb up and this is why we get the reputation as 'dangerous' during pre-menstruation – because if we are keeping a lid on our emotions, and our thoughts are in charge, stresses and dramas are much more likely to occur and we're much more likely to react OR become a ticking emotional time bomb.

Bitchcraft

Yep, bitchcraft is TOTALLY a thing. It's the refinement process and when I say refinement, it's NOT about taming your wild essence as a woman, but allowing ALL your feelings and emotions to be felt and present, and you to show up in your wholeness and then respond from a place of truth and knowing.

It's not a free pass to say whatever the hell you want and not worry about the consequences, it's an opportunity to trust that the signals, prompts and information you receive during the second half of your menstrual cycle are calling forwards what needs to be seen. They will show you where you're not taking a stand, where boundaries are being crossed, they'll show you what you need to let go of, what no longer serves you and ask to you to see and recognize what you have been too busy to see during the rest of the month.

If you DON'T pick up the messages your body sends you, those messages will show up as physical problems or they'll manifest in your outer life through a crisis or drama of some kind to get your attention.

During your pre-menstrual phase download after download is available to you, but if you don't slow down or create the space to unpack them, you'll miss them entirely. This is when PMT cramps and gnarly pain can manifest. PMT is an internal playback of the past days, weeks, even years of the things that need to be released, dealt with and healed. It can be a simple message that is urging you to slow down or a massive neon sign screaming at you to make changes in your life that could bring about a healthy balance physically, emotionally, and spiritually for you.

Only you know the answer to that, and you'll only ever find out if you do the freakin' work.

The flowing and swelling that occurs in the pre-menstrual phase is your body's way of bringing ALL of this to the surface and screaming: 'See me, listen to me, don't look away from me, bring me home, love me, heal me.'

This is how we become the wise women; this is how we fully embrace our SHE power. Ask yourself in each pre-menstrual phase:

- What is there for me to learn here?

- What does my current need to scream *really* mean?

- What can I learn from it?

- How am I not taking care of myself?'

But remember this is NOT the place to act on any of this. I encourage you to journal your entire pre-menstrual phase. From day 21 through to bleed, write down what's pissing you off, who's pissing you off, where you're not sharing your voice and where you're feeling frustration. I REALLY try to stay off social media during this time because there will always be a Facebook post that will tweak my nipples and send me spiralling – you've been warned. Hormone fluctuation during this phase means it's not the time to be having the BIG conversations, because while your no bullshit filter is on, your ability to speak with any kind of compassion is LOW, so any talking is best kept for the solar part of your cycle.

As you learn the messages of your body and begin to heed them, PMT will no longer be something you fear; instead it will become an insta-messaging service that allows you to reconnect with SHE and learn how to slow down, receive and take a big, deep exhale.

The more skilful we get at picking up our own signals, listening to our wombs and feeling our feelings, the more we can take action from a place of power. SHE power. This way, less drama and pain needs to show up for us to learn our lessons and we're able to:

- Take radical self-responsibility.

- Stop thinking that you have to fix everyone and instead tend to your own wholeness.

- Care less about what people think of you and allow yourself to feel and express. FULLY. (No matter how messy and intense it gets.)

- Create boundaries, learn to say no and stand up for yourself.

Basically bitchcraft is a chance to explore your natural instincts as a woman, those parts of you that don't belong to the people-pleasing good girl that patriarchy/society/your parents have told you to be. These wildly undone and untamable instincts are a universal wisdom that is innate to the feminine.

~ KALI BITCH, PLEASE ~

The following SHE Flow practice will allow you to work with the feelings that can emerge in this part of the cycle and to allow them to move through you and not try to escape from them. It takes the masculine energy that's created in the warrior yoga asana and makes it the dance of the warrior queen – RARRR! (You can watch an instruction video of this in the downloadable Lady Landscaping Toolkit, see page 251.)

You WILL feel fire. The fire will help you to let anger, annoyance or whatever you're feeling in the moment be there and felt. You can then use that fire if you so wish to alchemize those feelings through movement.

Fire starter

1. With your legs slightly wider than hip-width apart, keep your left foot facing forwards and turn your right foot to a 45-degree angle, stretch your arms out wide, keep your feet strong. Inhale, twist gently at the waist, so your torso is facing right.

2. Take your arms up to the sky and, on the exhale, bend forwards at the waist over your right leg. You don't have to touch the floor, just go as far as feels comfy. This will give your womb and belly a gentle squeeze and allow heat to build in your belly. See what needs to be seen and feel what needs to be felt.

3. On the inhale bring your arms above your head. On the exhale, bring your torso back to centre and your arms stretched out wide and away from your body.

4. Now repeat steps 1–3 on the left side.

5. Repeat this exercise five times and FEEL the fire.

Sword fight

1. With your legs slightly wider than hip-width apart, keep your left foot facing forwards and turn your right foot to a 45-degree angle, stretch your arms out wide, keep your feet strong. Inhale, twist gently at the waist, so your torso is facing right.

2. On the exhale grab hold of two imaginary swords and like a warrior queen, take them across the front of your body in a figure-of-eight. Keep your feet firmly rooted and do this for a count of eight.

3. On the inhale bring your arms above your head. On the exhale bring your torso back to centre and stretch your arms out wide and away from your body.

4. Repeat steps 1–3 on the left side.

5. Repeat this exercise five times and let the swords cut away anything that is no longer serving you – people, places,

situations. While doing this practice on the right side, you may experience masculine problems – the men in your life, authority, organizational and patriarchal issues – and the left side of your body may evoke feminine problems – friendships, misunderstandings and matriarchal issues.

RARRR!

1. With your legs slightly wider than hip-width apart, inhale, take your arms out to the side and bend them at the elbow so you're standing like an upright cactus.

2. On the exhale, bend at the knees, stick your tongue out, Kali Ma style and let out a breath, roar, scream whatever feels good. Let whatever is moving through you be released.

3. Repeat this exercise five times and then allow yourself to be still. Don't try to reach out or fix any of what comes up, let it rise, let it be seen, let it be felt.

~

The contraceptive pill

I had a MASSIVE revelation about how I was totally dishonouring my power as a woman by medicating my bleed.

Now, I'm no Judge Judy, so there's no judgement if you choose to use hormone-based contraception, but if you do, I urge you to hear me out.

Before I had a contraceptive implant fitted, I medicated my bleed for 15 years with a contraceptive pill that makes levels of globulin – the stuff that binds testosterone and affects our libido – four times lower, for ever.

If that wasn't scary enough, I had no connection AT ALL with my cycle because anything that pumps synthetic hormones into your body – the coil, implant, the pill – will affect your natural rhythms. As well as stopping you from getting pregnant, it creates a synthetic balance that numbs the ebb and flow of your cycle. Basically, if you're currently on the pill, that thing that you've been calling your period isn't one at all.

And what I know now, that I didn't know then, is that when you're not able to connect with your cycle, you're not connecting with your body and her true nature.

And when you don't connect with your body and her true nature?

Life goes to shit when we try to do it like a dude.

Taking the pill watered down my entire experience of being a woman – the cyclic ebb and flow of emotions, access to my super powers, the energies that are YOU-nique to each of us and become heightened at specific times of the month. As a result, I became totally numb and senseless to the wisdom my body was trying to share with me – so that I could mask the fact that I bled from both others and myself and could function more 'normally' in the world.

For normal, read masculine.

The pill silences our direct hook-up to our true nature, to our ultimate SHE power. We deny ourselves the opportunity to truly know, protect, claim and embody, and most importantly love, being a woman.

That PMT pain?
It's for a reason.

Your reaction to the coil or the pill?
It's a message from your womb.

I'm not a doctor, but if anything I've said causes a twinge in your womb, read *Sweetening the Pill* by Holly Grigg Spall immediately, and get all the information. If you need help making decisions about the pill speak to people you trust. My deal is that synthetic hormones numb your body from the female experience, and I didn't want to be numb to that anymore, so I stopped. Do I advise my clients not to take them? Well, the ones who want to get preggo, obviously, but the others, I tell them what I'm telling you: get all the information.

Pharmaceutical companies have a vested interest in telling people that birth control can preserve their fertility; my personal experience and that of so many of my clients is that it's part of the problem, not the solution. Talk to people you trust and figure out what's best for you because there's a best thing for every body.

The five best reasons to come off hormonal birth control

If you're considering coming off the pill or other hormonal birth control method, you might have been thinking about it for some time. Maybe you've done some research (thanks, Google!) and seen some stuff that's got you scared and apprehensive about taking that step (again… thanks Google). Maybe you're just unsure what you're going to do about contraception if you take that step. Whatever the reason for your decision, and there are many good reasons not to use hormonal birth control, you might be finding you're not getting a whole lot of support from your doctor, health practitioner, or even your partner and your friends.

MUFF MUSE - HOLLY GRIGG-SPALL

There are many great reasons not to use hormonal birth control and here follows my top five:

1. **You'll enjoy sex more!** *It's pretty much guaranteed that hormonal birth control has thrown cold water on your sex life in some way, at some point. Whether it's made you less interested in sex, reduced your sexy dreams, given you less lubrication, pelvic pain or a harder time getting orgasms. Taking a pill to prevent you from getting pregnant, which also then stops you wanting to even do the thing that might get you pregnant, is one of life's cruellest jokes on women. We think not having to worry about getting pregnant will be the most amazing aphrodisiac (it makes sense!), but these synthetic hormones have the effect of removing the libido peaks we would otherwise get with a non-medicated cycle. For many women, coming off the pill is a revelation. All of a sudden they really want sex, like physically want it, in a way that they may not have felt since being a teenager.*

2. **You'll improve your relationship.** *The body's hormones impact how we react to other people and how they respond to us. Many studies have shown that using the pill causes men to behave differently around women and skews how women feel about men. Some experts even recommend women try coming off the pill before marrying their long-term partner, just to check that they're really attracted to him. If you're single, you might find not using the pill helps you tune in better to your intuition when it comes to seeking out a date. If you're in a relationship, coming off might cure any doubts you have. Not feeling solely responsible for preventing pregnancy is also really important for*

some women sharing that part of a relationship can open you both up to more communication and intimacy.

3. **You'll experience all the feelings.** *Although the pill can help some women avoid the perils of PMT (that said, there are better ways…), many women decide to come off it because they feel it has caused them, conversely, to experience mood swings, depression or anxiety. The effect of hormonal birth control on your mood might be obvious to you now, or you might be questioning how it makes you feel after a decade or more of using it. For others, these methods of contraception cause a 'blah' or dulled-down feeling that means they find it hard to get excited or feel really happy or enjoy life to the fullest. Everyone's different. Going pill-free can bring in a whole range of feelings and mood changes – some women have said it's like coming out from under a cloud or from behind a veil. Colours are brighter, tastes better, and smells sweeter, a bit like when Dorothy switches from black-and-white Kansas to Technicolor Oz – but without the weird little wizard man.*

4. **You'll up your fitness game.** *This is a little-known fact unless you hang out with professional athletes – hormonal birth control prevents you from gaining muscle effectively. Some athletes have also noticed that the pill makes them retain water weight through bloating. This all links back to testosterone – the pill pretty much wipes out our testosterone levels, which we need for energy, sex drive, and for building strength and fitness. So, choosing non-hormonal birth control might help with your goal to tackle a triathlon this year or just to lose those surplus 10lb. At the very least, it might make it less of a drag to get to the gym a couple of times a week.*

5. ***You'll stop worrying about scary headlines.***
   Unfortunately, some methods of hormonal birth control cannot be categorized as safe. We're seeing more and more in the media about the blood clot risks associated with the pill and other hormonal methods such as NuvaRing, and that's because new brands with new formulations have been shown to have a significantly higher risk than the hormonal birth control methods of the past. You may have even already swapped your method because you read an article or your doctor mentioned the issue.

   As we get older our bodies change, we gain weight, we might be more sedentary – and as such our personal set of risks change. If the headlines have made you uneasy and you don't feel like you should be at risk of death just because you want to avoid pregnancy (especially when there are so many other options out there for you), then coming off hormonal birth control can be a big sigh of relief.

Bleeding in sync with the moon

Lots of women, when they find out how our cyclic nature replicates that of the moon cycle, begin to long for the days when we all bled together at the dark moon and ask how we can sync our cycle with the moon. There are ways, but for me, I'm concerned that women might use it as yet another stick to beat themselves with, as in 'I don't bleed with the dark moon, so I'm less in touch with Mumma Nature' – that kind of thing.

Not true.

My research has shown that your period will attune to both cycles of the moon, (dark and full and the times in between) over the course of your life, but it's fascinating to note what's going on in your life energetically as your body cycles.

So, what is your body trying to tell you?

If you bleed at or near the dark moon, you'll tend to bleed during the new or waning moon. Since biodynamics show that the earth is most fertile during the full moon (when you ovulate), this cycle is most traditionally linked to fertility and motherhood. You'll likely feel a surge in your intuition during your period, and will feel the urge to withdraw for nourishment and self-renewal. In other words, you're tapped out energetically and have given the month your all—it's 'you' time.

If you bleed at or near the full moon, this cycle follows the full moon, meaning that your body bleeds during the waxing or full moon and is most fertile during the new or waning moon. Full and waxing moon phase energies are outgoing, vibrant and creative so some feel this is counterintuitive to menstruation. Not so. In ancient times, this was associated with shamanism, high priestesses and healers. Women who tend to menstruate with the full moon are said to focus their 'darker' and more creative menstrual energies outwards, rather than inwards, in order to nourish and teach others from their own experience. Many times, women with this cycle will be more focused on self-growth, development, mentorship and creativity.

I'm sure it'll come as no surprise to anyone that during the writing of this book, I've been bleeding on or a day or two after the full moon.

But really, there's no right or wrong.

None.

This is ALL an exploration.

Cycle awareness

So, many us of don't know what a 'regular' cycle actually looks and feels like, because we've not been taught. Advertising teaches us to 'stuff up' our bleed with tampons and forget about it so we can 'carry on as usual' – partying, riding on boats and roller skating in white jeans – is shown as a 'normal' way to exist when it's anything but normal for most women.

Not everyone bleeds the same, not everyone's cycles are the same and how it is for me, is not necessarily how it'll be for you, which is why I'm really passionate about charting – not just circling the day you start bleeding in your diary (although that's always a really good place to start) but also charting your moods, your actions, your feelings and how you've showed up for yourself, in work and with your family.

Seriously, if I had been taught charting from my first bleed, I'd have had a go-to guidebook to my entire range of moods, feelings and emotions.

I would have had fewer arguments with my parents, I'd have had a better understanding of the dynamic in my friendships with ladykind and quite frankly, I'd have had a far, far better sex life in my 20s.

There is so much to be excavated, and it really is a lifetime's work but some of my favourite cycle findings have been in my relationship with the Viking. Now I crush on that hot hairy Viking lots, but there are times in my cycle when sex is not high on my list of things to do and I'd much prefer to curl up on the sofa and have cuddles. However, there are other times when I send him saucy texts at work and demand he comes home immediately.

There's a delicious intimacy that comes from understanding yourself and your sexual/romantic wants and desires (and sharing this knowledge with your partner, too). You may discover that during menstruation you need to pull away, or that after menstruation you need slower, more attentive loving, while at ovulation you crave more passion and energy and want it NOW. You may find that you're more sensitive in different parts of your body at different times in the cycle – maybe you love your nipples being tweaked in your late spring, but in your autumn phase? Not a freakin' chance.

Knowing all of this makes life as a woman so much bloody easier to understand. So share what you find out with your partner. Get them involved in the charting process, and most importantly encourage them to explore, experiment and get to know you and your body and your sexual preferences at each phase of your cycle with you. It really does make for an awesome relationship in and out, under and on top. See what I did there? THIS is how it is for the Viking and I. It's not perfect, far from it, but when we communicate with our partners, an understanding develops, a way in which we can navigate the lady landscape together.

And if you're in a same sex relationship, this is JUST as important if not more so, because you can't just assume that how you're experiencing your cycle will be the same as it is for your partner just because you're both bleeding women – for example your day 24 may be a shocker, while her day 24 is a day for deep introspection, so be sure to both chart and not to assume that how it is for you is how it is for your partner.

The reason I love this so much? Living in tune with each part of our cycle means that we give equal priority to all aspects of our life and ourselves. We naturally begin to meet our changing needs in each phase; we stop having unworkable expectations; we understand ourselves better; and we can begin to reduce the stress we place on ourselves to remain consistent.

Ah, let's all collectively breathe a sigh of freakin' relief.

What I share here are just brief snapshots of each phase and the power that they hold. Working with them is not a quick fix, in fact, nothing about ANY of this work I share in Love Your Lady Landscape is a quick fix.

NONE... OF... IT...

We live in a quick-fix society, where we take the pill, follow the diet, become famous by being on *X Factor*, but the whole ever-unfolding SHE quest of being a woman is cyclic. You're on a feminine journey that will take you deeper and deeper into who you are and will unfold medicine for you in each phase and with every cycle you experience. The quick fix is how ever long it takes for you to reach menopause, because it's only then that you can fully experience the wholeness of being a woman. So, just surrender to trusting that your body is wise.

Surrender to the flow.

Surrender to trusting SHE and the actions SHE leads you to take in response to your body's cyclic nature – it's quite the adventure!

The menstrual cycle as an initiation

I know this because my menstrual cycle prepared me for the death of my parents.

My mumma, who only had months left to live was very specific that the Viking and I go on a trip to Dubrovnik. I didn't want to leave her. I was in a constant state of waking up wondering if today would be the day she left her body, but she was adamant.

I agreed to go for a long weekend. I was bleeding, I was tired and run down and welcomed the idea of sun on our bones.

On the day we were due to leave, I received a message from a policeman that my dad had died. It was a shock. Totally unexpected. Having been so worried about my mumma dying, I was completely unprepared for my dad dying, too. But on my mumma's command, we still flew out to Dubrovnik in the afternoon.

Despite being a teary grief-stricken mess, we were upgraded to first class – the perks of being a Called Girl. SHE will always hook you up with what you need – and in that instance, I needed a glass of wine, a big seat and proper cutlery.

On arrival, Magdalene Travels arranged our transport. Of course it was. (Anyone who knows my back story knows that Mary Magdalene first appeared to me the day my mumma was diagnosed with pulmonary fibrosis – the sacred synchronicities and cosmic winks that have happened between then and now have been endless and plentiful – she truly is my home girl.)

We arrived at the hotel and were the only guests, so were given free access to all the spa facilities and a penthouse suite scattered with Magdalene rose petals. Our housekeeper introduced herself as Mary. After a deep and much-needed sleep, we headed into the Old Town. As you enter the walled city, there's a shrine to Mary that all the locals touch for luck. I gave her a li'l rub in appreciation for the cosmic winks she'd sent so far. Later in the day, after ice cream and lattes, we decided to go on a boat ride, as we climbed on board, the Viking gave me a nudge. The boat was called *Magdalene*.

When we returned from the boat trip, a tour bus had just arrived in town with over 30 people wearing badges with 'Magdalene' written on them... and so it continued for the entire three days – and we were upgraded on the way back, too.

When we arrived home, Mumma got really poorly and three days later, the Viking and I sang and chanted and cried with her, as she took her last breath and left her body.

My parents left their bodies within 10 days of each other.

It was an initiation.

There was so much fear, pain and grief, yet having a strong foundation in my truth, in my teachings, having firm roots in Mumma Nature and her cycles of death and rebirth gave me a strong resting place for the grief to come.

I knew that despite how much it hurt, if I stayed with it and let it move through me, 'this too shall pass'. My knowledge and my menstrual teachings gave me a pillow to rest on to allow myself to be transformed for ever.

My menstrual cycle was a beautiful resource that helped me to stay soft and connected to my body and feel it ALL. It was a surprisingly beautiful thing to stay in my centre, to not abandon myself and to stay connected to SHE and ALL her medicine at a time when I felt I was falling apart and never going to heal.

**When forced to face your biggest
fears – sit in your centre and heal.**

Celebrating the cycles of SHE (and life)

When we connect with our cyclic nature we deepen our roots into the truth of who we are and we awaken to the many faces of SHE. I am totally devoted to my menstrual cycle as spiritual practice – I'm a Called Girl, remember? It's what SHE called me to do. I wanted to be a fashion designer when I was a kid, at no point did I tell the careers advisor at school that I wanted to talk about lady landscapes and blood and guts and ancient women's medicine and wisdom.

There was definitely NOT a tick box for that job.

When I came home to myself through my menstrual cycle, I came home to Her. To SHE.

SHE started to speak to me through my cycle. Each phase is SHE in different forms and SHE is initiating us each and every month, in each and every phase.

It's also why I now take so much joy in celebrating the seasons of life as a celebrant and I adore creating contemporary rituals that tap into ancestral and cosmic wisdom, in a way that is relevant and accessible to women in the modern day.

I was blessed when I was asked to create a Welcoming Womanhood ceremony for my sister, friend and fellow Hay House author, Rebecca Campbell, in preparation for her marriage. Think super-spiritual hen weekend. While the contents of the ceremony will remain Rebecca's to share, I can tell you that when you fully welcome womanhood in sacred ritual, when you allow yourself to become a woman unto herself, your life WILL change.

In lots of cultures around the world, a girl's transition to womanhood is celebrated in ritual and ceremony; it's the time of coming into her creative and spiritual power, yet so many women in the Western world have lacked this celebratory entry into womanhood, and this has affected everything from their attitude to their menstrual cycle to how they view the body they currently reside in.

Our menarche, our first bleed, is when our song, our life purpose, our truth is awakened in us.

With each cycle we sing louder, speak truthfully and nurture that bud as we respond to, and work with, the lessons it provides, allowing us to open and grow into the wholeness of who we are.

Imagine if we had all known this, at that moment of our first bleed – how would it have been different?

For me, I'd have stopped trying so hard to be 'someone' in my late teens and 20s, because I'd have been able to trust that with each bleed cycle, life was unfolding me, just as it should.

There would have been flow – literally and figuratively, as I narrated the story of being this woman from a place of truth and purpose – my womb.

~ MENARCHE STORY ~

So, what was your first bleed like?

What did it feel like? Where were you? Was it celebratory? Was it negative?

I invite you to put yourself in that young girl's body, in that moment, right now and allow your heart to simply riff on it in your journal.

Depending on your first bleed experience, this may feel traumatic; or it may feel like a total non-event but know that your menarche story is a powerful insight into the woman you are now, so dare yourself to really go there.

If your experience was a celebratory one, how did that make you feel? To have the moment you became a woman, marked by family and friends? Were you proud? Were you embarrassed?

- If it wasn't celebratory, what was it like?

- How did it feel, physically and emotionally?

- Where were you?

- Did you tell your parents? What was their reaction?

Revisiting your menarche story is like a deep-dive self-excavation into who you are and why you do the things you do. This is your story, and to become yourself fully, you need to claim it. Share it with your girlfriends, share it with your partner, share it with your children. Share it on your blog or in a sister circle in person or online.

If, once you've started to revisit your menarche story, you don't like what you've discovered, consider writing yourself a love letter in that moment of your first bleed: tell her everything she needs and wants to know in that moment.

- What didn't she hear that would really have helped?

- Who would have spoken to you?

- Would they have hugged you?

- What would they have said to you?

This is something we are not traditionally encouraged to remember or celebrate, so I've created Red Reconnection – a biannual event in Mumma Nature. A place and time where women, who were not celebrated or honoured at their first bleed, can gather to receive a menarche ceremony and be welcomed into womanhood. If you're not able to get to either of these events, visit the website to sign up for the online Red Reconnection (see Resources, page 247).

~

This isn't a rewrite of your history, it's an opportunity to identify your feminine wounds and let the healing begin.

CHAPTER 5

Pelvic Power

*'Whatever you want to give birth to,
believe me, it will help if you reconnect
with the power in your pelvic bowl.'*
DR CHRISTIANE NORTHRUP

In the practice of SHE Flow, I help women to establish a solid presence in their root and make their medicine through regular 'down there' self-care.

Why is this so important? Because when you are present in the root of your body on a daily basis, you respect the ebb and flow of mumma nature, the seasons and your own body; you're able to experience connection and not separation and you can express and receive it all.

**Joy, pleasure, pain, light, dark,
creativity and nourishment,
SHE power fuels you.**

So, let's go there… Let's go 'down there', behind the flaps and let's really get to know your lady landscape.

I take Paloma the Pelvis to all my workshops. Paloma is a life-size pelvis with a removable colour-coded plastic uterus, bladder and anal passage. As I hand her around the circle and women poke around and see how everything fits together, they're mesmerized.

When I explain that our pelvis doesn't sit like a free-standing bowl, the same way that it does in a masculine body, and it tilts forwards (which is why when a yoga teacher tells you to 'tuck your tail bone under' it's actually not possible – grrr), I find them eagerly wanting to feel how it is for them, in their body.

Most – probably 95 per cent – of my clients come to me because something is wrong 'down there', yet for many of them, Paloma the Pelvis is the first time since that one class in biology, that they've seen what their pelvic bowl actually looks like and they begin to understand how it works. We shouldn't be waiting until it's 'broke' before we get educated, we need to become the number one authority on our body and we need to own our throne.

Your pelvis is your seat of power.
Queenie, it's time to own your throne.

Your seat of SHE power

Your pelvic bowl is the physical and energetic place within your body that holds feminine power, wisdom and medicine. It's your personal cauldron of lady magic. It's a BIG DEAL. Yet so many of us are numb to her existence. We don't know how she feels or what's she's trying to communicate to us unless she's screaming in pain – or in some cases, pleasure.

A Mayan priestess, a shaman named Rosa, described to me how in shamanic traditions, the pelvis is known as the 'second skull' so if you're experiencing tension in the jaw, it will be mirrored by tension in your pelvis – they are in an energetic relationship with each other.

Rosa is not a show-shaman with all the feathers and face paints. She's the real deal. She is a 40-something Italian who lives in a little house in France where she experiences the same every-day existence as you and I, but also with extraordinary access to the greatness of it, thanks to teachings that she's received from the Grandmothers of Guatemala.

I went to see Rosa after I'd split with the supposed-to-be-forever-love. Work was scarce, and I was experiencing pain in both my jaw and in my pelvis. When I described where the pain was she nodded and said, 'Your pelvic cradle – the central core of your being – is stuck, sore, painful and stagnant, yes?'

I wouldn't have put it *quite* like that, but it turns out that tension and misalignment patterns in the hips and jaw very often 'mirror' each other. So if your right side of the jaw is more tightly clenched than your left, then the right side hip muscles are often tenser than those on the left. Similarly, if the jawbone protrudes forwards, it is common for the pelvis to also be tilted or jutting forwards from its more normal, comfortable position – which was true for me – I had a protruding jaw and a tilted pelvis to add to my list of 'faulty' body parts.

Rosa reassured me that I wasn't faulty goods and explained how the ancestral, energetic and emotional imprints, which created this pelvic imbalance, had become more pronounced and painful, and that we attract 'accidents' or events into our lives that reinforce this pattern and make it worse.

Rosa is now a treasured teacher and after exploring my hip–jaw connection as a deep-rooted need to express myself both verbally and sexually – something I wasn't doing at the time because it was stuck, sore, painful and stagnant –she introduced me to some pretty amazing Mayan GG-mumma teachings. One of which involved her dry humping my womb for 20 minutes while listening to a pan pipes soundtrack and making me cry. (Ha! I assure you this is really an incredible technique called 'pulsing' and one that I now offer clients myself). Basically, the Mayan GG-mummas believe that the pelvic cradle is a sacred container of our Feminine Crown, which not only makes you the Queen (*own it, g-friend!*) but also means the subtler movements – sensitivity, touch presence, awareness, love, attention, forgiveness, gentle movement and breath – can bring the very deepest healing to this area.

Now ideally, the organs and muscles in the pelvic bowl would have good alignment; energy and blood flow would be strong and vital to enhances cellular health and hormonal circulation; and you would be in loving communication with it to guide your life and give expression to your creative dreams. I mean, that's the ideal scenario, but for most of us, it's uncomfy to drop our attention down to our pelvis – we have no concept of how our anatomy works, it's dark down there, it's damp and sometimes it's bloody.

But deep within your pelvis you hold wisdom and the ability to create – not just babies but ideas, projects, dreams, desires and urges – and when you connect with your seat of SHE power, you begin to cultivate a real feminine presence. It takes the term 'feel-it-in-your-body-ment' to a whole new level. When your SHE power – your energy and essence – becomes embodied in the pelvis, it's magnetic. You live from your true centre and life flows to and through you. You begin to feel a powerful, enchanting energy awaken and unfold inside you, a force field which is pulsing, alive, dark, rich, creative and fertile.

Before I share some Mayan GG-mumma practices for you to try yourself, I'm going to talk about the physical terms of the structure of the pelvis and the reproductive/fertility system, so that when we work, touch and feel her, we can visualize where different parts are and recognize where emotional and physical tension, pain or numbness show up. So grab an 'I heart my lady landscape' mirror and pull back the flaps for SHE anatomy 101. Because we need to know exactly what's in there, how it works and what lady magic we can make with it, right?

SHE anatomy 101

The softness and the receptivity of the female anatomy has been celebrated, admired and subjected to abuse, violence and mistreatment over the millennia. Author and activist, Eve Ensler, has led a movement of women who now speak openly about the true nature of female sexuality thanks to the *Vagina Monologues*, but despite the countless features online and in magazines dedicated to a woman's 'sexual satisfaction', very few of us really know any deets about 'down-there'.

I know that I was embarrassed when I didn't know that a uterus and womb were the same thing. Forget that – I wasn't embarrassed, I was annoyed.

Annoyed that I had to go and get trained in pelvic healthcare to learn about my lady bits.

Annoyed that a disturbing number of women are having surgery to have a 'designer vagina' or removing their 'down-there' hair because they feel pressurized by what porn/men/society have decided how a vulva should look. (*They're all totally and gloriously different, BTW.*)

Annoyed that I would go into schools to teach sex education and wasn't allowed to encourage 16-year-old girls to explore their vagina, cervix and labia lips with their fingers, so they knew exactly where they were and how they felt, because when we know that our female anatomy not only serves a physical purpose but also has potent energetic SHE medicine to share, it's vital that we know how to access it.

The following will make much more sense if you look at your 'down there' with a hand mirror while you read the text. Make sure you have enough time and privacy to feel relaxed. Try squatting on the floor and putting the mirror between your feet. Oh, and download the SHE anatomy 101 colour-in sheet (part of the Lady Landscape Toolkit download, see page 251) (*Yep, I've drawn you colour-in lady parts – what's not to love about that?*)

Also, for the lady-part geeks, if you're after super-science-y explanations, head to page 247, where I share some of my favourite resources. (*I'm a total geek too, so I hear you, info-seeking sister!*)

What I share here are the basics, and I take a much more psycho-spiritual approach to make our SHE-scape as easy to understand as possible, so science talk is kept to a minimum, 'K?

Read my lips

Pussy, va-jay-jay, lady garden, vag, bush, beaver, fanny, muff, the notorious V.A.G., Lawrence of a Labia, Mary – what do you call your lady parts? Our place of pleasure, our genitalia, our vulva, our clitoris, our vagina really has been, until now, the area that shall not be named and by not naming it, we're basically saying it doesn't exist. Personally, I use both cunt and the Sanskrit term, *yoni* (pronounced *yo-nee*), which means sacred womb space because I think it sounds sensual and love-filled, and that's how we should feel about this sacred place in our body. If we don't name it something we love, how on earth can you show her love or expect others to love, respect and honour her either?

We have very limited language to describe our sacred body, least of all loving and sensual language, and it's up to us to change that and to challenge it in others. Otherwise adverts that shame our yonis and vulvas – think feminine wipes and deodorizers – will continue to perpetuate the myth that there's something wrong with us and that we're not worthy.

Your yoni is perfect. It looks perfect, smells perfect and can cause you to feel perfectly wonderful things. It can be waxed, shaved or plucked, or it can be left in its perfectly lovely untouched natural state.

It's your property. I recommend respecting her, only sharing her and loving her on your terms. Explore your own cultural beliefs regarding lady parts and bleeding. Look at the words, language and phrases that are currently used to describe her, pay close attention to the advertising of feminine hygiene products – how do they make you feel? If certain words make you cringe or balk, dig around and find out why? Maybe your mum didn't like it and that dislike has been passed down to you. Perhaps there's shame and embarrassment attached to a certain phrase or word.

I was literally struck mute when I first heard the word 'cunt'. I found it vulgar and harsh, that the idea of using it as a loving word wasn't an option for me, but as I got familiar with its origin, I began to practise saying it, I'd try it in different accents and with a smile. I began to say it internally while lying in *shavasana* at the end of a yoga class and holding my hands in a yoni mudra (see page 42) and slowly, it's become a word I love.

Naming her, talking about her with love and affection, honouring her as sacred will allow you to start trusting her as your guide, letting her inner wisdom move through your entire body. The same will happen when you embrace your cyclic nature – when you ritualize your menstrual cycle and live day to day in a more ecstatic way, you will become enriched by ritual and flow and as a result, you'll become more intuitive, vibrant and satisfied.

You will claim your worth as a woman, and damn it woman, you are SO worthy.

Vulva

Your vulva is the outer part of your lady landscape and that includes your clitoris, labia lips, urethra and entrance to the vagina. In Sanskrit, the vulva is called a yoni, which means 'a divine passage way' or 'temple doorway'. The vulva opening is almond-shaped, which in sacred geometry is called the *vescia piscis*. Its outline is formed when a circle passes through the centre of another, creating between them a two-pointed oval – an inter-dimensional doorway. Basically, our vulva, our yoni, is an energetic gatekeeper, that can help us to understand what we want to bring in and what we want to release.

Clitoris

Your clitoris is awesome and the only organ in the body with the sole function of providing pleasure. Oh yeah.

When people talk about the clitoris, they're usually just talking about the glans – the very sensitive outside part, but the bean-like bump you can see on the vulva is just the tip of an iceberg.

The internal part is connected to the glans by two spongy areas of erectile tissue. Further down, it branches off into a pair of wings that extend into the body and around the vaginal canal like a wishbone. Then, underneath are the clitoral vestibules, or vestibular bulbs. Like much of the clitoris, these sac-like structures of tissue become engorged with blood when you get aroused.

It's the most nerve-rich part of the vulva containing over 8,000 nerve endings – twice as many nerve endings as the penis – making it the powerhouse of pleasure. *Just saying.* This tiny erogenous zone then spreads the feel-good-love to 15,000 other nerves in the pelvis, which explains why it feels like your whole body is being taken over when you orgasm. (For more about how to stimulate see page 202.)

Labia

Your labia are the lips that help protect the clitoris and the openings of the vagina and the urethra. The labia majora are the outermost lips and the labia minora are the inner lips. In some women, the labia minora are completely hidden inside the labia majora and not visible externally, in other women they protrude – both lip situations are perfect and completely normal.

Unfortunately due to pornography showing women with hairless vulvas and all the lips tucked neatly inside, some women feel embarrassed or ashamed of their natural and completely healthy variations, and turn to plastic surgery to get a 'designer vagina'. This can lead to the loss of sensation and pleasure in the entire area, which personally, is not a risk I'd EVER be willing to take. The 'average' labia lips are 2–10cm long, yet most of the labia lips shown in pornography are virtually invisible.

All labia lips – chubby, big, hidden, lippy, thin and lovely are all normal and glorious whether tucked away or wanting to be seen. In his book *Yoni: Sacred Symbol of Female Creative Power*, Rufus Camphausen explains how the classical sexologist texts of India – *Kama Sutra*, the *Ananga Ranga* and the *Koka Shastra* – use the type of lips and the love juices they produce to read the psycho-physical make-up of a woman. Brings a whole new meaning to the phrase 'read my lips', doesn't it?

Urethra

Located between your clitoris and your vaginal opening, this tube leads from your bladder to the vulvar vestibule (the area inside the inner lips of the vulva where the vagina is) and carries urine out of your body from your bladder.

Vagina

Your vagina is not really penis shaped, it's a pulsing muscle that opens and closes, and is the muscle between the cervix (at the base of the uterus) and the external opening from which babies and menstrual blood can exit and into which fingers or a penis can enter if you choose.

Perineum

Your perineum is the outside of your urethra, vagina and their attached muscles. However when we refer to the perineum we tend to think specifically about the bit of skin from the bottom of the vagina to the anus, the bit that may feel good when it's touched during sex.

SHE TRUTH

If you're finding it difficult to take a look 'down there', check out beautifulcervix.com – a website that celebrates the beauty and intricacies of women's bodies and fertility. Women submit photos of their cervix during the menstrual cycle, pregnancy, after termination, and after orgasm. You can also view photos of a cervical (pap) smear test in progress, too.

The internal lady landscape

The uterus, ovaries and fallopian tubes are located between the bladder and rectum in your pelvic bowl.

Ovaries

Your ovaries have two main reproductive functions in the body. They produce eggs (called ova) for fertilization and they produce the reproductive hormones, oestrogen and progesterone. My most favourite fact to share about the ovaries is that we have all of the eggs we're ever going to have when still a foetus inside our mumma's body.

Think about that for a minute.

On a cellular level, you actually existed in your g-mumma's body when she was pregnant with your mumma. It also speaks to how deeply and energetically connected we are as women and how, and why, we unconsciously hold our mumma and g-mumma's energetic patterns and beliefs in our own body. It's why when we connect with our seat of SHE power we can transform this energy from our family lineage. We can heal our mumma wounds.

The left ovary is feminine and controlled by the right side of the brain and its energy is receptive, creative and intuitive, while the right ovary is masculine, controlled by the left brain, and has more of a 'doing' linear energy.

Fallopian tubes

There are two fallopian tubes and they take it in turns each month to carry the egg (ovum) from the ovary to the uterus. A section of the tube, the ampulla, is generally where a man's sperm fertilizes the ovum. The resulting zygote (fertilized ovum) then moves to the uterus where it implants in the uterine wall and continues to develop until birth.

Uterus or womb

The uterus has three layers:

- inner lining (endometrium)
- middle muscular layer (myometrium) – the strongest muscle in the female body because it assists with pushing the baby out of the uterus during labour, fact fans
- outer layer (perimetrium)

The uterus is like the wise woman that all the other organs gather around deep inside your body and is composed of:

- fundus – the dome-shaped section at the top
- body – the central juicy bit
- cervix – which opens into the vagina

The uterus is our centre of creativity and intuition – the place where all life begins. If you conceive a baby, the uterus is where the baby is grown and nurtured. If there is not a baby in the womb, this space is pure creative potential. Anything that requires imaginative energy – business plans, relationships, writing a book – can all be birthed energetically from the root of your womb.

Psoas muscle

An important and often overlooked part of the pelvic bowl is the psoas muscle (pronounced *so-ass*), which extends from the spine through the pelvis and into the top of your legs. When this muscle is strong and supple it helps us to be juicier In our passion for life, allowing more Shakti to flow through our system.

I am obsessed with the work of Liz Koch. Liz knows EVERYTHING about the psoas muscle and wrote *The Psoas Book*. SHE Flow consists of a lot of hip opening movement with the specific intention of releasing tension in the psoas and hip flexors, because when you relax your psoas, you literally energize your deepest core by reconnecting with the powerful energy of Mumma Earth.

Liz believes that our fast paced modern lifestyle chronically triggers and tightens the psoas – when we stress or get tense, the muscle contracts and eventually shortens. This can lead to painful conditions including low back pain, sacroiliac pain, sciatica, disc problems, knee pain, menstruation pain, infertility and digestive problems. A tight psoas muscle can also constrict the organs, put pressure on nerves, interfere with the movement of fluids and impair breathing. In fact, Liz says,

> *'The psoas is so intimately involved in such basic physical and emotional reactions, that a chronically tightened psoas continually signals to your body that you're in danger, eventually exhausting the adrenal glands and depleting the immune system.'*

Which is why when we look to cultivate a healthy medicine bowl of lady magic, we have to pay attention to our psoas. Our modern lifestyle is restricting our natural movements – sitting at desks for hours at a time, the position of car seats, wearing constrictive clothes and high heels (I know this won't be popular, but wearing heels can throw your whole pelvic bowl out of alignment) – and so a constricted psoas muscle equals heightened nerves, high adrenal levels, pain and dis-ease in your medicine bowl. Not cool.

**A released and relaxed psoas lengthens
and opens, it wants to dance, it conducts
energy; it grounds us to the earth
and allows the spine to awaken.**

Liz says,

> 'As gravitational flows transfer weight through bones, tissue,
> and muscle, into the earth, the earth rebounds, flowing
> back up the legs and spine, energizing, coordinating and
> animating posture, movement and expression. It is an
> uninterrupted conversation between self, earth, and cosmos.'

Basically, it's a freakin' lightening rod connecting you, Mumma
Earth and SHE – let's look after it, yeah?

～ SHE Flow:
Shakira-Shakira hip openers ～

This exercise is attributed to the great songstress Shakira
because you can't do any kind of hip opening practice without a
little Shakira-Shakira love.

In SHE Flow, I rarely suggest holding a pose, but what follows is
the exception to this rule. It's a 35-minute yin-inspired practice
for really gently stretching into the deep connective tissue of the
body and bringing love and connection to your psoas muscle and
pelvic bowl.

Yin yoga is a slow-paced style of yoga with poses – asana – that
are held for long periods of time (five minutes or more). I'll be
honest – at first I didn't love it, which FYI is generally a sign that
you need to at least pay attention to why you don't love it. This
particular practice offers deep access to the hips and pelvis, and

the time spent holding the postures is much like time spent in meditation – an opportunity to breathe into the medicine bowl, to activate and open it and bring energy and vitality to it. As always with ANY energy or movement work in this area, it can create space for emotions to come to the surface – fire, anger, tears – this is why I didn't love it initially. It brings up 'stuff'. But let it. Let it all be there, and let it move through you throughout the practice.

1. Roll out your yoga mat and sit comfortably.

2. Bring the soles of your feet together, making a diamond shape with your legs in front of you.

3. Inhale, reach your arms above your head and bending at the hip, exhale and take your arms down to the floor in front of you. Take this stretch as deep as feels good for you without pushing yourself. Now breathe. Follow your breath and let gravity pull you down towards Mumma Earth, not your muscles. Now hold it here for 3 minutes. You can pulse slightly with your breath, letting gravity pull you deeper.

4. Inhale and slowly walk your hands towards your body, lift from the hip and return to sitting position with an exhale.

5. Inhale, place a hand under each knee and on the exhale, slowly and gently, guide them towards each other and place the soles of your feet on the floor.

6. Inhale and as you exhale, gently lower your body back towards the mat.

7. Inhale, take your feet off the mat and bring your knees towards chest into a foetal position. Hug them here for a while and rock from side to side giving your lower back

a gentle massage. (If you have a tilted pelvis or a big bum like me, this can feel a little uncomfy, so don't be afraid to adjust until it feels good – we're only interested in it feeling good, OK!)

8. Place the soles of your feet on the mat, bend your knees and, keeping your bottom on the floor, inhale and, on the exhale, allow both legs to drop slowly to the right side of the mat. Feel the stretch over your left hip. Activate your feet by pointing your toes towards your knees (this gives the knees some protection). If this is too tight, bring your heels closer or further away from your bum. If it's not enough, put your right leg on top of your left and breathe here for three minutes.

9. Bring your knees slowly back to the middle, placing both feet on the mat. Windscreen wiper your knees from side to side slowly three times. Inhale, keeping your bum on the floor as much as you can, and, on the exhale, drop your knees slowly to the left. Again, if it's too tight adjust the distance of your feet from your bum. If it's not enough, then place your left leg on your right. Activate your toes and feet towards your knees and breathe deeply while you hold it here for three minutes.

10. Bring your knees slowly back to the middle, placing both feet on the mat. Windscreen wiper your knees from side to side slowly three times.

11. Keep your right foot on the mat and bring your left ankle to rest on your right thigh. Put your left arm through the hole made by your legs, and the right arm down your right side and connect your fingers under the thigh of your right leg. Inhale and lift your right leg from the floor.

Activate both feet by pointing the toes on each foot toward the knees. You can make this stretch deeper by pushing your left elbow in towards the right knee. Now hold and breathe deeply for three minutes.

12. When complete, unfurl your left leg, stretch both legs and point the soles of your feet towards the sky. Keep your left foot on the mat and bring your right ankle to rest on your left thigh. Put your right arm through the hole made by your legs, and the left arm down your left side and connect your fingers under the thigh of your left leg. Inhale and lift your left leg from the floor. Activate both feet by pointing the toes on each foot toward the knees. You can make this stretch deeper by pushing your right elbow in towards the right knee. Now hold and breathe deeply for three minutes.

13. Unfurl your right leg, stretch and point both the soles of your feet towards the sky. Bend your knees towards your chest, inhale and grab the outside of your feet, your soles facing the ceiling. Exhale, drop your knees as wide as they'll go and feel the stretch. Breathe here for three minutes.

14. Stretch your legs up and point both soles of your feet towards the sky. Inhale, bend your knees, bring your soles together, exhale and make a yoni shape with the arches of your feet. Inhale, grab the outside of your feet-yoni with both hands and exhale bringing it to face level, so you can see through your foot-yoni. Breathe here for three minutes.

15. Inhale and on the exhale, drop your feet to the mat, stretch your legs out in front of you and your arms over your head – stretch, stretch, stretch.

16. When you're ready, give yourself a well-earned 15-minute Yoga Nidra (see page 210) while in *savasana* – your pelvis will thank you for it!

~

Connecting with your medicine bowl

Knowing about your anatomy isn't enough. You need to feel it. Feel what you're holding on to and what can be released.

I place my hands over my womb space every night before I go to sleep. I take some deep womb breaths and take a few minutes to tune in to the flow of Shakti in my centre. I feel her, I talk to her and if, for some reason, I feel a cold or numb sensation over my womb then I gently focus my attention on it until the energy begins flowing to that area. Sometimes, if I'm holding on to a thought or belief, or I'm feeling anxious or tense, it'll be harder to create an instant flow, so I'll rub her or give her a womb massage (see page 164). This simple practice lets her know she's not being ignored, that you love her and brings you back to your SHE power – and creative potential – that is your birth right.

How it is for you, will be different from how it is for me, because our pelvic bowls all contain different medicine for our SHE quest, our life ahead. It's a bowl of possibilities – pleasure, pain, power, periods, pregnancy, potency, penetration and it's up to us to make it a moment-to-moment practice to connect with her and seek her counsel.

One in three women are raped or sexually abused and this can cause the power portal to shut down. We disconnect and unplug from her because we think she's spoiled, and we carry that shame and blame around with us. When we can start a conversation with her, when we can send love and kindness, we can lift the shame and we begin to make the world safer for everyone.

∼ TUNING IN TO YOUR MEDICINE BOWL ∼

To tune in to the energy of your medicine bowl, gather some paper, pens, cushions, a yoga mat and a music-playing device and come down onto the floor for this three-part exercise.

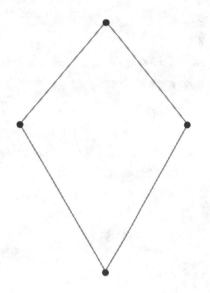

Example yoni map

Yoni map

We're going to map your yoni. (*Yep, that's exactly what it sounds like.*) Don't worry you don't have to get naked. Unless you want to, obvz.

1. Take a piece of A4 paper and sit on it with your legs hip width apart in front of you. Move from side to side, until

you're sitting comfortably on your sitting bones. Bring the soles of your feet together so that they're touching in front of you. Don't let this be painful, put cushions under your knees so they're not under any strain.

2. Take a pencil and run it down the front of your pubic bone and make a mark on the paper.

3. Now things start to feel like you're playing a game of solo-twister with yourself, especially if, like me, you've got a tilted pelvis, feel where each sitting bone lands on the paper and make a mark either side.

4. Once you've done that, reach behind you and where your anus is, make a mark there.

5. Take the paper out from under you, and you should have four dots that, when joined together, create a diamond shape. This is your yoni, your sacred temple gateway. Place her in front of you, bring the soles of your feet back together, sit upright with your head over your heart and your heart over your womb and breathe. (Sit on a cushion for this if it's more comfy for you.)

Stirring the cauldron

I do this in every SHE Flow class because it activates the entire pelvic bowl area and brings any medicine to the surface that needs to be experienced.

1. Put on a song you love – I recommend *Returning* by Jennifer Berezan for this – get comfy and drop down into your body. Feel the physical sensation of your sitting bones, allow your breath to move your energy down into your pelvis.

2. Now, keeping your knees still, begin to slowly make small circular movements with your belly and pelvic bowl.

3. Depending on how you're feeling, begin to take your circles wider and wider.

4. Allow your arms to reach up above your head or sit on your knees – whatever feels good.

5. When you feel like your cauldron is fully stirred, change direction coming slowly back in towards your centre, until you're barely moving at all.

6. When you come to a stop, place hands palms up on your knees, and breathe.

7. Sit quietly for a few minutes and feel.

8. Place a hand on your womb space and ask her:

    ~   How do you feel?

    ~   What texture are you – soft, hard, spiky, smooth, silky? How are you moving – pulsing, thrashing, moving in waves, still? What mood are you in – angry, sad, joyful, happy, minxy?

    ~   What colour are you?

    ~   What do you want to be called?

Make yoni art

I now invite you to get creative and allow your SHE medicine to guide you in making a piece of art from your yoni map dedicated to how your yoni feels.

Maybe you want to write her a song or a poem, cover her in glitter or put a lightening strike through her to represent her power. Maybe you want to colour her all black and place barbed wire around her or gather material based on the textures that she described to you and craft a sensory experience. The only rule is to create a piece of art that represents her personality and essence and your relationship right now. When I first did this, I did it in each phase of my menstrual cycle and it was so powerful to see how my relationship with her and her personality changed with each phase.

If playing solo Twister with yourself to create art isn't your thing, use the questions above as journal prompts, or download the SHE anatomy colour-in sheet from the Lady Landscaping Toolkit (see page 251) and use the questions to prompt you as you colour in. No one's judging your art, what's important is that you're connecting with the wisdom, guidance and clarity that can be found in your very own medicine bowl.

Gather your friends, do it in a circle, share stories, frame it, put it on your altar.

If you're called, I'd love for you to share your yoni art on social media, with the hashtags #loveyourladylandscape and #shepower – you don't have to tell people what it is if you don't want to, but I just love the idea of my Insta-feed being filled with literal lady landscapes.

~

This is a public cervix announcement

You might find that connecting with your womb and medicine bowl proves tricky if it's pissed. And let's face it, if you live a fast-paced modern life, if you medicate your menstrual cycle, if you sit down in an office or drive a car, if you're not aware that your rhythms and cycles are your direct connection to Mumma Earth, there's a REALLY good chance you'll have a pissed-off pelvic bowl.

According to statistics published by the World Health Organization in December 2012, there is an epidemic of infertility and 'down-there' dis-ease: it is currently experienced by over 7.4 million women in the Western world with approximately 85–90 per cent of that dis-ease being treated with drug therapy or surgical procedures.

SHE TRUTH

I meet the majority of my clients when something has gone wrong and 'modern medicine' is not working for them. At the SHE clinic, I work practically and psycho-spiritually with SHE Flow massage and movement, therapy, ritual and embodiment practices to help women access their body wisdom to heal their pelvic bowl health, so please know that what I'm sharing here isn't to scare or worry you, it's to stop women's health issues going unnoticed.

Women have a baseline expectation that we're supposed to have pain. We literally accept that being in a lot of pain is what we have to 'endure' as a woman. We think that heavy painful periods that interfere with school/work/relationships are normal and we get fretful that we'll be judged as 'weak' if we admit to pain. And then there's delayed diagnosis from medical practitioners who have limited time and resources and 'generally' work on a process of elimination when dealing with 'down-there' care – which is frustrating for them, but even more frustrating for us, so the most important step in taking care of 'down there' is to educate yourself.

What's 'normal'?

Waxing and access to porn means we're definitely aware of what's 'down there', but it also means we have a slightly warped idea of what's normal. As I described earlier (see page 132), the vulva is one of the most variable parts of the body with many, many different versions of 'normal'. It changes appearance throughout the menstrual cycle, so if you've still not looked at yours, put the book down, go get that mirror and get familiar with the messages your body and your lady landscape is sharing with you each and every day – fluid changes, textures, colours. The following are all normal changes.

- Just before your period, your genitals can become a little swollen and a bit lumpier.

- Skin cysts can also appear and also can get bigger and feel a little sore at this time.

- Things also change, as you get older. Sex and birthing babies can make the inner labia lips stretch, and weight loss and gain can affect the appearance of your lips, too.

- After a vaginal birth, things will definitely feel and look different. Don't be afraid to feel around, the inner labia lips may look a little different and may hang when previously they didn't, or they may not.

- There are lots of colour variations, too.

- Your vagina makes mucus 'discharge'. In menstruating women, vaginal discharge has its own 'cycle', with not much just after a period, very clear and stretchy mucus in the middle of the month, and then getting heavy and thicker as the next period approaches. The colour can vary from clear to almost yellow.

CH-CH-CH-CH-Changes

But changes in the area should never be ignored. Here's what to look out for and when…

Discharge

Vaginal discharge is normal and will vary with age and throughout your menstrual cycle, but if it smells, causes itching or is a colour other than clear, white or off-white, it *may* be a sign of an abnormality. These symptoms can be a result of thrush, which is due to yeast that lives naturally in the vagina and can produce a thick, white discharge that may smell sour and itch a bit.

See your medical practitioner if it doesn't improve within a week, as it may be another issue like bacterial vaginitis (BV) or a sexually transmitted disease (STD).

Never ignore blood outside your period. While this can occur if you've changed contraception or are on the mini-pill, always see your medical practitioner, as it can be a sign of an STI (sexually transmitted infection), damage to the vagina or, in very rare cases, cancer.

Smell

We each have our own smell, and you only need to be concerned if it becomes more noticeable. A fishy odour with a grey, watery discharge can be a sign of BV. Good and bad bacteria live in the vagina, kept in balance by levels of acidity. If something changes that acidity (such as sex or using soap) a bad bacterium, called *gardenerella*, can flourish, causing symptoms to occur.

Lumps and bumps

A bump that's always been in the vagina or vulva is probably normal, but new lumps could be a result of genital warts – which can be singular or appear in clusters.

A lump under the skin is more likely to be a cyst in the Bartholin glands, which secrete lubrication during sex, and if it gets blocked a painful lump forms. I've had a few of these and they're ouch-y.

In both the above cases or, if you're not sure then always see your medical practitioner for advice.

Colour change

The vaginal area is normally a colour similar to the inside of your cheek. This can change during pregnancy. The most common reason behind colour change is irritation, which will make it angry and NO ONE wants an angry vagina, right?

Thrush can be to blame but washing powder, bubble bath, or even dyes in your undies – cheap black knickers may contain a substance called paraphenylenediamine in the dye – can all trigger an allergic reaction.

What's not normal?

With each vulva having it's own unique-to-you muff-print, it's impossible to give a comprehensive list of what isn't normal and how to detect it, but I want to share some super basic information about some specific 'down-there' discomfort and dis-ease that women can experience and how they effect the reproductive organs because…WE… NEED… TO… KNOW…

Cervical cancer

The second most common cancer in women worldwide develops in a woman's cervix (the entrance to the womb from the vagina). It often has no symptoms in its early stages. If you do have symptoms, the most common is unusual vaginal bleeding, which can occur after sex, in between periods or after the menopause. Attending your regular screenings is vital in detection and prevention.

Fibroids

Benign (non-cancerous) growths can occur in your womb (uterus). Most women have no symptoms while others may have painful or heavy periods. If they push on the bladder a frequent need to wee may occur. They may also cause pain during sex or lower back pain. A woman can have one uterine fibroid or many of them.

Endometriosis

In this condition, tissue, which behaves like the lining of the womb (the endometrium), is found in many different areas of the body, including the ovaries and fallopian tubes, outside the womb, the internal lining of the abdomen, the bowel or the bladder.

Endometriosis is a long-term (chronic) condition. Symptoms can vary significantly from person to person, and while some women have no symptoms at all, others can find themselves experiencing painful or heavy periods, pain in the lower abdomen (tummy), pelvis or lower back, pain during and after sex, bleeding between periods, difficulty getting pregnant. Most women with endometriosis get pain in the area between their hips and the tops of their legs. Some women experience this pain all the freakin' time. Basically it sucks and how severe the symptoms are depends on where in your body the abnormal tissue is, rather than the amount of tissue you have.

Endometrial cancer

Arising from the endometrium (the lining of the uterus or womb), this cancer is the result of the abnormal growth of cells that can invade or spread to other parts of the body. The first sign is most often vaginal bleeding that's not associated with a menstrual bleeding. Other symptoms include pain with urination or sexual intercourse or pelvic pain. Endometrial cancer occurs most commonly after menopause.

Polycystic ovary syndrome (PCOS)

This condition affects how a woman's ovaries work. Cysts develop in the ovaries (polycystic ovaries) and so they don't release eggs regularly and high levels of 'male hormones' called androgens are found in your body.

Polycystic ovaries contain a large number of harmless cysts up to 8mm in size. The cysts are underdeveloped sacs in which eggs develop. In PCOS, these sacs are often unable to release an egg, which means that ovulation doesn't take place.

Symptoms of PCOS usually become apparent during late teens or early twenties and can include: irregular periods or no periods at all, difficulty getting pregnant (because of irregular ovulation or failure to ovulate), excessive hair growth – usually on the face, chest, back or buttocks, weight gain, oily skin or acne.

Ovarian cancer

This disease can disrupt the normal function of the ovaries. If left unchecked, it can affect other parts of the body, too. Ovarian cancer occurs when abnormal cells within the ovary start to multiply, creating a tumour. But it's important to note that not all tumours are cancerous. Ovarian cancer symptoms may range from nothing at all to a persistent stomach pain or bloating, finding it difficult to eat or feeling full quickly, needing to wee more often.

For anyone who follows me on Instagram or has met me in person, you'll know that I'm probably the most obsessed with vags/pussies/lady landscapes hetero-girl you'll ever meet. I've been scraped, I've had smears and scans, I've had laser surgery on my ovaries – and the more I connected with my upset uterus and what was going on physically and spiritually in my medicine bowl, it became infinitely interesting to me, which is why I now love that I get to talk to women about their bodies, their muff musings and their healing.

These are the conversations we should ALL be having, because when we don't, women's health issues go unnoticed. Pay attention to your body, chart your menstrual cycle (see page 90), touch yourself, look at your vag in a mirror and learn what's normal for you. That way you're more likely to notice if it changes. If something worries you, you can go get it checked out because you're not embarrassed by her. When you care for her, you care for you.

Fierce-ass warrior and amazing friend, Diane Evans is currently undergoing treatment for ovarian cancer. Her story, her pain, her healing is for her, for you and for me.

MUFF MUSE - DIANE EVANS

When I was diagnosed with ovarian cancer I was advised of the extensive surgery I would require, which included removing my womb and both ovaries. I know many women have gone through this before me but the prospect began to hurt my heart, throwing me into a deep, dark hole.

I had always wanted more than one child and I am truly blessed with his life, but I also experienced waves of regret and remorse that I lost two babies and had always yearned for more. Feelings of fear bubbled away inside of me, burning into my sad and now redundant womb like a hot knife. I felt the hard lump of grief already coiling round and round in my solar plexus making me feel sick to the core as so many emotions surfaced that I hadn't expected. I felt too weak to deal with the deep emotions this invoked, but there was no choice but to face it head on.

I sought advice from several female friends who had experienced a hysterectomy, but for every view and piece of advice that was so generously shared, it was their journey and experience, it wasn't mine. I had just under six weeks until my surgery was booked and this gave me a chance to dig deep and find my way through and to recover from the initial exploratory surgery that led to the cancer diagnosis. This proved to be incredibly valuable time for me in that I had anticipated my grief and I could start cutting the ties with my womb before she was removed from my body. I desperately wanted my womb returned to me following surgery, but this was not possible due to the disease in my abdomen, so holding a funeral type ceremony for my womb in which she could be returned to the Earth was denied to me.

In the weeks leading up to the surgery I tried to get my head around what would be left inside of me after all my sacred lady parts had been removed – I couldn't visualize the empty, raw and disfigured space at all. I struggled to imagine my beautiful sacred womb space without my womb being in there and started to cut the ties with my physical womb, rather like psychic surgery I guess. In a meditative state I gently wrapped my beautiful womb in a soft shroud of love and gratitude for all that she had provided for me in my life as a woman and I started what was to be a regular process to let her go with my blessing before the surgery took place. I did not want to think of my precious womb being coldly removed from me by a surgeon who just could not have an understanding of my deep spiritual connection to her, so I chose to take on that role myself. What would soon be an empty womb space, I filled with a rich, vibrant and golden light leaving the empty space sacred and whole again. With incense ingredients I made a mandala-type image of my altar at home to represent my physical womb, which I needed as a tangible way of believing this was happening.

Alongside this process of letting go I wrote words that came to me through meditation: deep, heartfelt, emotional words that fully embraced all that I would have said during a funeral ceremony to offer my womb back to the Earth. Despite being prepared physically for the ceremony, I couldn't bring myself to let go completely at that point. It took another two months after my hysterectomy for me to feel ready and I share with you the following words and rituals I used in a womb-cutting ceremony:

'I call upon the Goddess Cerridwen to stand with me and guide me as I prepare to cut the emotional ties with my physical womb. I ask that her wisdom teach me how to make the transition from the Mother to Crone phase.

'My physical womb will be taken from me on the 1st April and I release any emotional ties to it with my blessing, gratitude and love.

'I honour all that my womb gifted me as a Maiden and Mother and I give thanks for my dear child who grew within my womb and marvel at how my body could have created such a beautiful being.

'I give thanks and am in awe of all that my womb taught me as a woman and that its sacredness remained intact even when my deep feminine core was undermined.

'As my physical womb is taken so, too, will the pain it has held on to at the sight of red and the deep primal scream as my spirit children left my pregnant body. It was not their time, but I remember them and love them always even though I carry the grief of their loss within my heart.

'I let go of the pain of failed relationships and events that left deep scars within my sacred womb space and give thanks for the lessons I learned because of them.

'As my physical womb has served its purpose and is now a potential danger to my life I cut the emotional ties I have with it and allow it to be taken with dignity and grace from my body.

'I open my sacred womb space so that it can be filled with a rich, healthy, vibrant golden light. My spiritual connection with my sacred womb space pulsates with life and I embrace all that the Crone phase brings with deep love and gratitude.

'Cerridwen, I give thanks for your presence, your guidance and your wisdom as I join the millions of women in this phase of my life.

'I let you go with my heartfelt Blessings.'

I also went on a meditation journey with the beat of my trusted drum. I followed a path at dusk that led me through lush green grass to a forest. Following the path I eventually came across a fire in a clearing where a group of unclothed ladies were gently swaying to the drumbeat. They were all crones of many more years than me. One lady with long silver hair took my hand and I recognized her as Cerridwen. She guided me through cutting the emotional ties with my physical womb.

With my eyes closed I laid down on the warm grass beside the fire and felt my physical womb letting go of my body and move through the birth canal until I could feel it with my fingers. I picked up my dying physical womb and cradled it in my cupped hands and stood to offer it up to the Gods. I swathed it in black cloth and scattered rose petals over it before placing it in the flames of the fire. Swirls of smoke rose up into the darkening sky and I wept as I watched my physical womb return to the Earth. I gave the ashes of my physical womb back to Mother Earth, giving heartfelt thanks for all that it had gifted me and acknowledged the pain it had held on to for too long.

Finally, to let go in the physical realm, I waited for a waning moon before grinding and then burning some of the incense in my cauldron from the altar mandala that represented my physical womb. As I did so, I read the words out loud that I'd written for my tie-cutting ceremony. Then I folded up the piece of paper on which I'd written my words and burned that with the incense in the cauldron.

For now I feel I have done what I can to prepare my physical womb for its removal.

I give thanks for my beautiful and sacred womb space that will always reside within me for it now has a different meaning and a different role for me in life.

Letting go of my womb was the beginning of the process, and it is truly a process.

Following Diane's hysterectomy, her sister Julie unfortunately had to have one shortly after, too, and she requested for her womb to be returned. The surgeon had never been asked before, but high fives to him for genuinely listening to Julie's feelings and taking her request seriously and for returning her womb following surgery. However, it took a lot of persistence and form filling but Julie was determined – love that! She purchased a small, beautiful, ornate wooden box to hold her sacred womb safe for burial, and she wrote a ceremony similar to one you would use at a funeral. She took a close friend with her to a special place that she visits in a local woodland, and she held her sacred ceremony there.

Her words gave thanks for all that her womb had gifted her throughout her life; the potential, her sacred femininity and the joy of all that being a woman brings. Julie had always wanted to birth a child but for many reasons, this was not to be. She read her words of remorse, regret and apologies for not gifting her womb the opportunity to hold a child in her sacred space and shed tears of sadness and grief. Julie gave her womb back to Mumma Earth with reverence and has a special place to visit, too.

Two journeys, two sisters, two healing paths.

**Let's pause and take a deep breath
and give big love to our wombs,
our sisters and Mumma Earth.**

CHAPTER 6

SHE Care for 'Down There'

'The feminine spirit of the jungle reminds us of this simple and vital truth: The womb is not a place to store fear and pain; the womb is to create and give birth to life.'

MARCELA LOBOS

So let me gather together some of my favourite ways to care for 'down there' and yes, I'll definitely include the Guatemalan G-mumma technique that Rosa did to make me cry, too – it's pretty special. And funny. And sacred. But mostly funny, then emotional and then special again.

Rites of the womb

The Rite of the Womb, the 13th Rite of the Munay-Ki, honours the 13 moons of the year and is a contemporary ritual, birthed into being by Marcela Lobos, a medicine woman initiated in the healing and spiritual traditions of the Amazon and the Andes. The Munay-Ki are a series of rituals brought to the West by Marcela's husband, Dr Alberto Villoldo, distilled from his work as a medical anthropologist with the high shamans of South America:

> 'The rites of the Munay-Ki are based on initiatory
> practices of the shamans of the Andes and the Amazon.
> They are stripped of all trace of the indigenous
> cultures they come from. I did this to respect the native
> traditions, and to avoid the idea that persons from the
> West can become traditional shamans or Indians.'
>
> ALBERTO VILLOLDO, RITEOFTHEWOMB.COM

I received the Rite of the Womb while writing this book, in a gorgeous yurt called the Red Hearth on a Gloucestershire hillside in the UK. As soon as I received the rites, I knew I would be giving them to many, many women. Marcela expressly created this rite to be shared freely and urges you to go back to your communities and share the rite with others. I just love the simplicity of it.

There are very few words, paired with a very simple set of movements, but even now, as I grow and nurture the seed that was planted during my rite ceremony of smoke and sage and story sharing, I feel it's power.

I recommend this rite for all women, regardless of whether you are menstruating and especially if you have experienced hysterectomy, endometriosis, and/or any other surgery, ailment, or trauma of the reproductive organs.

SHE Flow womb, belly and abdominal massage

Belly rubbing and massaging was practised in the Egyptian temples of Isis, by Mayan g-mummas, Ayurveda practitioners in India and Norse goddesses alike to relieve any congestion or blockages that stopped the flow of energy and fluids of the circulatory, lymphatic and nervous systems in both men and women.

I received (and still do) womb massages to break down some of the painful endometriosis scar tissue that was causing me pain and to help me connect with and love my womb. I cried a lot because it's not just a practical, make-you-better therapy, it's a really beautiful, emotional healing modality too, which is why I trained in it so that I could offer it as part of the SHE Flow experience.

SHE Flow womb, belly and abdominal massage is an external, non-invasive massage specifically for fertility, menstrual and abdominal health, and it can also be used to correct the position of a uterus, too.

SHE TRUTH

Many women have a 'wandering womb' and don't even know it. Car accidents, overstretching during pregnancy or labour, running on concrete, chronic constipation, high-impact activities like dancing, aerobics, horseback riding, or gymnastics, wearing heels – can all cause your womb to wander.

Massage, pulsing and Rebozo shaking can all help strengthen the ligaments and muscles that support the uterus and ovaries. The combination of the massage, Rebozo and shamanic practices can also help to:

- Reconnect to the womb after trauma.

- Ease the pain and discomfort of menstrual health issues like endometriosis, PCOS and fibroids.

- Heal sexual health issues.

- Overcome fertility problems.

Basically, belly rubbing is goooood!

My teacher and mentor in womb massage is the amazing Clare Blake, creatrix of fertilitymassage.co.uk, but there are several versions of abdominal and womb therapy available worldwide. They are all very similar, so don't get too caught up about the differences between them. SHE Flow massage, Fertility massage, Mizan massage, abdominal sacral massage, Maya massage all draw on traditional techniques from different parts of the world, yet all are similar in the conditions they treat.

My advice would be to worry less about the name and more about your connection with the practitioner, their style of practice and their ability to serve your specific needs.

MUFF MUSE – CLARE BLAKE

A fertile womb is a creative womb, and I believe that, to heal the womb, is to heal the woman.

Fertility Massage blends womb massage, pulsing (a rocking Tai Chi style of bodywork) and Rebozo (ceremonial wrapping). Physically, the woman is nurtured, circulation to the reproductive and digestive systems is increased, and the fascia that holds the body tight, is gently rocked and released, allowing freedom of movement within.

Emotionally, this therapy gives women permission to reconnect to their bodies, releasing trauma, tension or shame and finding their inner womb wisdom.

Fertility and the desire for a baby isn't just about getting physically ready for motherhood, but we also need to be spiritually and emotionally open to welcome the new little soul. This was my original calling to this work, to help the souls waiting to come to parents that were ready. Along the way, the therapy evolved and I realized that the true depth of this work is about all women reconnecting, to enable them to feel empowered, inspired and creative.

I absolutely LOVE my work, it's like my own form of meditation, as I dance and move with my client to massage them back into their bodies. I use journeying with many clients to alter energy shifts, and this is not only powerful for each client, but I get to experience it with them, it's truly magical!

I equally LOVE teaching the massage to other therapists. When I see a room full of women blossom over our four days together, I know that the healing that takes place is not only within them but it'll impact their families, clients and communities. I get so emotional knowing that this is what I get to call my work. It brings me so much joy and wombtastic happiness sharing my gift, my blessing, my passion for Fertility Massage with so many women.'

∼ SHE FLOW WOMB AND BELLY MASSAGE ∼

I invite you to use this self-massage technique as part of your own love-your-landscape practice. It brings fresh blood and energy to your womb and digestive organs, it helps to realign your womb, releases any stress or tension and can help dissolve any emotional blockages you might be experiencing, too. It's also just a really bloody lovely thing to do each day to bring love and attention to your womb and medicine bowl.

Caution: Don't do this practice if you have an IUD or coil of any type, if you're pregnant, if you think you might be pregnant or if you're on your period.

Before starting, empty your bladder and create a quiet and cosy environment where you can relax for 5–10 minutes – just before you go to bed is great. You'll also want to be wearing loose and comfy clothes with no zips or buttons over your belly.

Lie on your back and place a pillow under your head and another under your knees to soften your abdominal muscles. Breathe deeply and slowly for a few moments until you feel relaxed.

Be gentle with yourself, use slow strokes and, if it doesn't feel good, don't do it! If you find areas of tenderness, pain or congestion, adapt your pressure so that you can continue to relax. Breathe and continue to massage the area. If pain persists, even with a light touch, stop for now. If you experience pain initially, it should gradually diminish with each self-care massage.

1. Warm your favourite oil or balm and make slow and large clockwise circles moving in the direction your digestion flows through your colon. Starting from your left hip, move up to the rib cage, under the rib cage and back down to the right hip. Do this three times, adding more pressure with each circle.

2. Gently, using small circular clockwise movements, massage across your lower belly, from hipbone to hipbone.

3. Place your fingertips in the middle of your upper abdomen on your ribcage. As you press here it will feel tender.

Gently come off this point and you will feel a dip. Take a breath in and on an out breath, press as deep as feels comfy for you into the soft tissue space and slowly move your fingertips toward your belly button. Repeat this three times.

4. Now move your fingers to just below your left ribcage. Take a breath in and as you breathe out, gently massage across diagonally across towards your belly button. Repeat three times.

5. Now move your fingers to just below your right ribcage. Take a breath in and, as you breathe out, gently massage diagonally across towards your bellybutton. Repeat three times.

6. When you've finished, gently place your hands on your lower belly, just below your belly button, and close your eyes.

7. Feel your SHE power under your hands and send your womb space love and gratitude.

8. Afterwards make sure that you drink plenty of water to hydrate your body and support the healing process. Thank yourself for taking the time out to take care of yourself today. You rock.

9. Honour your experience by paying attention to the changes and responding with what you need. For example, write your feelings in your journal or diary or share them with a trusted friend or therapist.

Repeat the self-care massage every day except the three days prior to, during your period, and the three days after.

~

Womb pulsing

So, the Mayan GG-mumma practice that made me cry is called 'womb pulsing'. Now, this practice is also said to have originated from the lineage of pre-patriarchal Tibetan Womb shamans, known as Khandros, who used the practice to awaken the SHE essence and the pulse of Shakti within us. What I know for sure is that ancient g-mummas from around the globe knew the best way to access suppressed energy in our womb space, so I'll share with you what I've been taught and how I share it with clients and we'll pay homage to ALL the lineages of ALL g-mummas that have ever been. How about that?

When Rosa shared it with me, we had previously had a conversation regarding suppressed orgasmic energy – basically, I hadn't had an orgasm that hadn't been clitoral-stimulated by me – so she had me lie on the floor, on a sheepskin rug in her treatment room and she instructed me to breathe deeply into my womb space.

I did this for 10 minutes, while she sat beside me with a hand on my womb and breathed deeply, too.

Then – and this is when it got interesting – she straddled me.

I *did* know she was going to do it, but all my thoroughly British hang ups instantly rose to the surface as this fierce Italian medicine woman hit play on the panpipes soundtrack, sat astride my womb, and began to rock gently back and forward.

Once my initial hang-ups subsided, and I was able to bring my attention back to my womb, I could feel Rosa's focus and intention there, too, and tears began to flow. I sobbed.

I sobbed for the disconnect, for the longing of deep from-the-core orgasm, for the need to be safe.

While listening to pan pipes, I came undone.

Rosa kept her attention on my womb and rocked, she'd change

the pace of her rocking being led by the energy of my womb. I sobbed (and laughed when bubbles of British embarrassment would work their way through me every so often) for 20 minutes, which is when Rosa came to a slow stop and climbed off my womb, sat beside me and let me be with me. In all my messy, tear-stained undone-ness.

The pulsing practice opened me up to receive, to feel and to allow. It did not however, make me love listening to pan pipes.

The process is done fully clothed and the pulsing itself moves stagnant energy that's stored deep within the womb space upwards in a spiral, so that it can be released. It's why laughing and burping and crying and screaming are all perfectly normal. The movement helps release energies from past sexual relationships, emotional trauma, energy imprints, clearing of ancestral baggage and removes stuck life force. By connecting vital points on the bone structure, feeling the pulse and the use of sound vibration, you can stimulate a positive energy current to flow through the womb space, discharging areas of pain and suffering that's stored in the nervous system.

I recommend finding a practitioner who can really honour your healing process, but don't underestimate the power of tuning in to your own womb, putting the SHE power playlist on shuffle for three songs, placing your hands about three fingers below your belly button, applying pressure (although not when you're bleeding or pregnant) and rocking her up and down gently to the songs and rhythms that show up for you.

~ OVARY BREATHING ~

Your ovaries are a powerhouse of creativity and when they're nurtured, fully charged and circulating with energy, you can use that SHE power to choose what you want to create and how to express that power in your body, through your body and then out in to the world. Connect with your ovaries and you connect with your ability to express yourself. Oh yeah.

The following exercise will help to awaken the creative powers of your ovaries.

1. Sit comfortably on a meditation stool or mat and place your hands over your ovaries – just below and on either side of the belly button – point your fingertips down towards the pubic bone, thumbs gently touching together near the belly button, creating an upside-down triangle over the ovaries.

2. Rest your tongue gently on the roof of your mouth, make sure both your jaw and your pelvis are relaxed and begin breathing deeply, in through your nose and out through your mouth.

3. Now, focus on sending energy to your ovaries, feel the energy expand and the warmth develop under your hands. Enjoy the rhythms and movement, say a mantra here, perhaps 'I am a creatrix, I am flow'.

4. Keep breathing into your ovaries and imagine a continuous flow of yellow energy moving in and around each of your ovaries and into the womb space.

5. While you are focused on the space under your hands, listen to your inner wisdom and allow whatever visions, feelings or emotions that surface to flow through you.

6. Be loving and be accepting of whatever comes up. If your heart starts to hurt or your throat becomes sore, move your ovary-made energy with intention to that area and use the out breath to exhale and clear what's stuck and no longer needed.

7. Allow the yellow light and warmth of the ovary energy to fill your whole body with creative potential.

8. Do this for as long as feels good to you. I recommend making it a lovely 15 minutes ritual at the full moon (if you'd prefer to make it personal to your cycle, don't do it at ovulation as your ovaries are already super-charged and stimulated, do it during your pre-ovulation or pre-menstruation phase) to really honour their ability to create and manifest.

9. When you're finished send your ovaries thanks and love and bring your hands into prayer at your heart. You might want to keep a journal close by as creative ideas and cosmic winks will definitely want to make themselves known!

After practising ovary breathing regularly, you will bring a lot of energy medicine to your ovaries, so expect to feel more creative and fertile in all the ways. Basically, be aware of your capacity to create – babies, magic, relationships, projects. With great ovarian power comes great responsibility.

Act accordingly.

~

Boob power

I can't talk about Lady Landscapes and not talk about boobs.

In their natural state, our breasts sit either side of our heart and they're a sensual, delicate and sensitive external expression of our heart energy. They're meant to move as we walk, it keeps the lymph moving and energy flowing, but many of us wear super-pretty but tight/underwired/push-up bras for 12 or more hours a day, and this can block the energy flow to our breasts and in some cases, can stop the supporting tissue growing all together. I go bra-less as often as I can, but if you're currently giving me the sly side eye at the idea of not wearing a bra indefinitely, whenever you can, free the boobies.

If you do wear a bra for long periods of time, making breast massage part of your weekly self-care routine can really help to show your boobies some love. Tantric practitioners in India have performed breast massage for centuries and its benefits include:

- relaxes tightness and tension
- sexual arousal
- soothes pain, soreness and discomfort
- harmonizes hormones
- flushes out toxins that can be stored in fatty tissue
- increases energy flow
- drains lymph, which helps prevent cysts, lumps and bumps forming

Regular breast massage can help balance the female endocrine system as well as cultivate sexual energy, and it's a great way to keep an eye (or rather a hand) on your breasts for changes or irregularities, too.

~ BREAST MASSAGE ~

I prefer to massage my breasts in the evening as it stops me from holding on to any stresses I may have experienced through the day, but you might dig a boob massage first thing in the morning, in the bath, after a shower – whatever feels good, do that. Your boobs will feel different during each phase of your cycle, which is why I recommend making it a weekly practice so that you can experiment with different touch and pressure.

You can do this standing or sitting up straight. Doing 36 repetitions of the following massage is recommended for increased energy flow and sensitivity, but I find counting makes the whole experience a whole lot less sensual and enjoyable, so you might want to do what I do: choose a 3–4 minute song that you love, hit play and let the music guide you.

1. Warm a couple of drops of rose oil (it shows big love to your heart chakra, see page 180 for more on the chakras) in your hand together with a generous amount of coconut oil.

2. When both hands are fully covered with warm oil, bring them to your heart. Take three deep breaths into the heart space before placing a hand on each breast.

3. Lightly rub in upward and outward circles. Your right hand will be moving in a clockwise direction while your left will be going anti-clockwise.

4. Let your hands move together up the inside of the breasts towards your chin, then outwards, downwards, inwards and upwards again. Don't hold your breasts and move them, but lightly skim the surface of the skin.

5. Change up the rhythm, move between a lighter and firmer touch, use your fingertips to smoothe and stroke the breasts, starting at the nipples and making spirals outwards.

There's no right or wrong way to do this – maybe you will come up with a breast rub all of your own. As with everything I suggest, just do what feels good.

~

Heal yourself, heal the world

Most of us are not taught how to clear out emotional baggage from trauma, abuse, day-to-day, toxic emotional experiences and ancestral lineage energies. If we embrace our emotions with each experience that we have, we can allow what we feel to pass through our bodies and not to be stored in them.

When we heal ourselves, we heal the wounds of the feminine – of our lineage, the women who have gone before, our sisters, and our communities. We don't have to hold on to the same story – we can rewrite it. In fact, it's our job to. It's why we're here – to uncover our wounds, name them and begin to look for ways to heal. When you get to know your lady landscape, when you begin to feel what's right and wrong, and trust that feeling, you can begin to send her love and kindness, and so heal your womb space.

**Remember don't go with
the flow, you ARE the flow.**

LADY LANDSCAPING TOOLS

SHE medicine

- **Pay attention to your SHE-scape.** Get to know what phase the moon is in and also what day of your cycle you're on (there are great moon calendars and cycle charts available – check out the Resources on page 247). This awareness will help you to gain a deeper understanding of yourself – physically, mentally and spiritually, so you can optimize your monthly super powers in work, relationships and. . . well, life.

- **Begin your rewilding.** Each waning moon/pre-menstrual phase of your cycle, explore the rage, the bitchiness and the wildness and let it be felt. The more it's allowed to be seen and expressed, the more you'll be able to speak and live your truth.

- **Own your throne.** Get familiar with 'down there' by taking a look and knowing what's 'normal' for you in your seat of power.

Mantra

Repeat this mantra any time you need a reminder:

'I surrender to the flow'

#BLOODYCONVERSATION STARTERS

These can be used as journal prompts, dive deeper questions, book club or SHE circle themes or, y'know actual bloody conversation starters on social media, with your g-friends or a stranger on the bus. . .

- What is your favourite season and how does that correspond with how you experience that season in your menstrual cycle?

- Describe your yoni in five words.

- What would it be like to fully trust and nourish your pelvic bowl and the medicine and wisdom that she provides?

Read

Joan Borysenko, *A Woman's Book of Life*

Stephanie Demetralopoulos, *Listening to Our Bodies*

Holly Grigg-Spall, *Sweetening the Pill*

Liz Koch, *The Psoas Book*

Lisa Lister, *Code Red*

Dr Christiane Northrup, *Women's Bodies, Women's Wisdom*

Lara Owen, *Honouring Menstruation*

Alisa Vitti, *Womancode*

Naomi Wolf, *Vagina*

PART III

LOVE
YOUR LADY
LANDSCAPE

Love the landscape
and terrain of your body
and love the
woman who
lives in there.

Chapter 7

Big-time Sensuality

*'Touch was never meant to be a luxury. It is a basic
human need. It is an action that validates life and
gives hope to both the receiver and the giver.'*
Irene Smith

There's a silent epidemic.

After menstrual issues, the biggest concern women have is that they don't feel sensual, sexy, empowered and horny.

Now this can be due to practical things such as taking the pill and/or antidepressants, but there's also societal, patriarchal, spiritual, energetic pieces at play, too, because not having a connection and reverence for our lady parts means SHE power, our vagina, our womb, our cyclic nature, our lady magic – EVERYTHING suffers.

The dude-centric world we live in means we have to constantly remember how to receive and to allow in order to fully respect and honour ourselves enough to explore our desires and pleasure.

THIS is the work.

But seriously, it's the BEST work and you don't have to do it alone – although the self-nourishment practice (see page 193) is definitely something you will want to try out solo – mmmmmmmm! The more we talk about how much sex we're not having and how many orgasms we're really faking because quite frankly we're shattered/our adrenals are mashed/our schedule is too full for pleasure, the sooner we can start to see where we're not showing up for ourselves, reconnect and live from a place of pleasure because it really is possible, I promise.

We don't realize how much is absorbed through our sexual centre. I believe that every person and thing that touches us intimately leaves an imprint – lovers, one-night stands, doctors, people who we didn't want to touch us, uncomfortably tight knickers, and even the cycle seat in spin class. (*I only went once, hated it!*)

Guilt, fear, shame, abuse can all get stuck in our womb space and create sexual organ armour. This is great at protecting us from the pain, but also stops us from feeling the good stuff. It can also creates all sorts of physical, emotional and energetic symptoms:

- repressed anger
- depression
- blocked sexual and creative energy
- frustration
- bloating
- fear of intimacy and abandonment
- low self worth/esteem
- unworthy feelings

So one of the most important lessons to learn on the love-your-lady-landscape adventure is to receive.

To fully receive.

I go into schools and colleges to talk to girls about self-esteem, body image, sex education and EVERY time we talk about sex, self-respect and the act of receiving, girls believe — yep it's really part of their belief system — that they should be the one giving pleasure, not receiving it. And when I ask them why they give pleasure, they say it's to receive love/validation/proof of existence and worth.

'If I give him a blow job, he'll like me.'

'He'll like me even more if I swallow.'

I'd sound the 'this-is-bullshit' horn, but honestly? This just makes me sad.

It makes me sad that I'm STILL hearing this from both women and girls.

It makes me sad that the ready availability of porn on the Internet means that many boys have a false perception about what women really look like.

It makes me sad that they might buy into the belief that every woman's prime goal is to satisfy his sexual needs by performing reverse cowgirl with body hair removed to within an inch of her life with absolutely no concern as to how to give her pleasure. (And for her not to love herself enough to know what she likes because she's never been taught to receive pleasure, and if she does know, not to have the confidence to ask for it.)

It makes me sad that there are women in the world who still haven't experienced an orgasm.

It makes me sad that some women will never experience an orgasm because their culture dictates that their clitoris is removed.

Loving my lady landscape is a daily practice in:

- Reconnecting with my body through movement and touch.

- Remembering who I am underneath the armour – a goddess, a priestess, a witch, a healer and a daughter of the Great Mumma. (A daily practice because no one wants us to remember THAT kind o' power.)

- Reverence for the incredible power portal that lies between my thighs. I worship, cherish and lavish my yoni with love. I chant to her, I breathe into her, I respect and honour her and all that she represents to me as a woman in the world.

- Receiving love and respect from my hot Viking husband who, at times, represents the patriarchal constructs that my Shakti, my divine female essence, often finds painful to navigate and negotiate. Yet he truly worships at the altar of SHE in me, tirelessly and without question, which allows me to receive the lessons, the pleasure, the grit and the blessings that being truly in my SHE power offers up.

Chakra khan

There are seven main chakras in the body – actually there's a WHOLE LOT more than that, but the most talked about are the seven that allow energy to run through the centre of the body. In fact, right now as you're reading this, your chakras are whirlin' and swirlin', expanding and contracting and responding to every little thing you're thinking, feeling, sensing, emoting, touching, seeing and tasting, both consciously and unconsciously.

Now, this isn't a chakra 101, (if that's what you're after, I'd totally recommend *Eastern Body, Western Mind* by Andoea Judith), this is a whistle-stop tour of your two lowest chakra centres, root and sacral. Both these chakras are located in the medicine bowl and it's where we hold on to and store some of the big stressors like anger, resentment, rejection, blame, shame, guilt, fear, intimidation and lack of self-worth, which is why...

> **EVERY woman should have an intimate relationship with the root and sacral chakras – the energy in their medicine bowl.**

If not acknowledged, we can allow some pretty gnarly programming to take up residence in this space and it will – consciously or subconsciously – come to the surface. Thoughts like:

- 'You're useless.'

- 'You're a bad girl.'

- 'It's naughty to eat that.'

- 'You can't make money.'

- 'You're worthless.'

- 'Who do you think you are?'

Feel free to add all the negative beliefs you have ever had about yourself to this list but these thoughts will ALL make themselves heard. And if you're not able to witness and recognize what they are and exactly where they're coming from in your body, they WILL have a negative impact on your self-worth and self-esteem.

So now it's time for me to introduce you to these two power points in your medicine bowl and the ways in which you can use them to reconnect with your body and yourself.

Root chakra

The root chakra name in Sanskrit is *muladhara*, and is located at the base of your spine and home to Ma Shakti – the very essence of life power. It's our foundation, how we ground ourselves and how we connect with Mumma Earth. It's commonly associated with basic survival instincts, like the need for food, water, a roof over your head, work, self-preservation and physical identity. It's where life begins.

When you trust life, you take good care of your body and your home, you feel calm, stable and grounded and keep a clear head, and your root chakra will spin beautifully. If not, then you may experience physical symptoms such as lower backache, colon issues, constipation, sciatica, osteoporosis, central nervous and lymph system, bone, adrenal and nail issues.

How to connect with your root chakra

However you do it, get on, and in, the earth. Really feel it, and don't just stomp over her unconsciously. Find time to be in nature, daily. Treat your body with love, nurture it, nourish it, honour it. Feed yourself fresh good food and drink lots of water. Get a foot massage. Take time each day to check in with your body.

My gorgeous friend Maya Hackett, creatrix of empresstides.com, takes barefoot medicine walks in nature daily, which is her way of exploring her relationship with nature, and helps her to listen to her instincts, let go of the worries and concerns of the day and be in the moment – each moment. So good.

**Do anything that will help you
come to know, really know, that
you have a right to be here.**

Sacral chakra

The sacral chakra's Sanskrit name is *svadisthana* and it's located just below your belly button. This is the energy hub for your emotions, sexuality, sensuality, pleasure, abundance and creativity. It reflects how you relate to yourself and to others, and plays a fundamental role in your intimate relationships. This chakra is a powerful doorway into the unconscious because it's where we harbour our deepest feelings.

When you refuse to let the media, reality TV or fashion magazines define what is beautiful or sexy, and instead delight in your body, dance, move, stretch, wiggle and moan with delight, your sacral chakra will fire on all cylinders. If not, you might not trust your creative abilities or worse you might even – consciously or subconsciously – sabotage your most creative ideas. You might also have difficulty reaching orgasm – no matter how hot and heavy sex gets, but may be too embarrassed to talk about why.

Basically, you'll feel a big disconnect from your carnal nature. This may show itself physically through gynaecological and sexual issues, yeast infections, low libido, STDs, ovarian cysts, endometriosis, bladder, pelvis and fertility problems, and menstrual cramps.

How to connect with your sacral chakra

Notice when your emotions ebb and when they flow, and who or what is around when it happens. Question yourself on a daily basis by asking questions, such as 'Why did I have that argument?' 'Why didn't I speak your truth?' 'Why did I suddenly feel happy or sad?' Holding on, repressing and blocking emotions denies their natural flow and healing qualities, and can eventually make you sick. If you can't speak your truth, write it down.

Write what you feel, feel what you write and do it often.

Don't be afraid to ask for help if you sense you need a little sexual healing, as the chances are your second chakra will have been through a LOT. For example, it may have been stuffed with lots of confusing and oppressive beliefs, everything from patriarchal religious views of female sexuality being dirty and unholy, right through to the 'perfect' portrayal of female sexuality in advertising that leads many of us to believe that our very worth is completely dependent on our beauty and how sexually attractive we are to others. Mix this with your upbringing, schooling and any past life 'stuff' you may have going on and you've a got a veritable sexual minefield burning in your lower belly – ouch!

I've called in NLP (Neuro-Linguistic Programming) practitioner, Kate Taylor of upcoaching.co.uk to help you ignite the wild colours of your root and sacral chakra.

MUFF MUSE – KATE TAYLOR

The first two chakras of the human body, the root and sacral chakras, connect us to the very core of our divine essence and all the realness that brings. They are both the seat of our very gravitational attachment to the Earth and all its power, as well as the centre of our relationship to self and the world around us.

We can often feel the most disconnection from these chakras as they are the furthest away from our heads. They move the slowest, so it's not surprising that we pay more attention to the upper energy centres – especially if we're head dwellers like me. I mean, it's exciting to want to develop your psychic abilities through your third eye intuition or to open the channel of your crown chakra so you can bring in the realms of beyond. In our world of seeking answers and quick fixes, it can be all too easy to pay attention to the upper half of our energy and forget that the lower half even exists.

Exist they do, and they do such an important job that we need to show them some love. Root and sacral are the caregivers of our body – the wisdom-keepers of our very souls. These babies move slow and deep and with real feeling, so they should be honoured with the same kind of care and attention they provide for us. There are no fast cures here; this is a life-long relationship of honour and respect – a time to reconnect with the generations of your lineage and an opportunity to tune in to everything deep within. There's rich beauty, essence and divine colour deep within each of us.

ROOT

Partnered with the crown chakra you can use the energy from both your higher self and your innermost consciousness to send down to your root. Sit with your bottom connecting to the ground and your tailbone as centred as it can be. Focus on your crown and send the energy connecting in from the top of your head down to your root. Bring the energy of the earth up through your tailbone to meet at the root chakra. Feel the warm glow. Imagine red warmth and energy swirling in and around the chakra as it vibrates and turns. Send deep slow breaths down and into the chakra, and with every inhalation send the affirmation 'I am grounded, I am peaceful, protected and secure in my essence. I bring the power of the earth into my being.'

SACRAL

As the sacral is all about relationships and intimacy with our self and others, it's time for us to become bonded with this energy zone. It's also our zone of creativity and joy — there's so much we can gain from working on this area — all we need to do is show some love.

This chakra's spinning partner is the third eye chakra, so you can allow your intuition to guide healing by tuning in to what she wants. Imagine that she has a voice within your body; what would she be telling you that she needs? What does she want you to know? This may take some time as it may have been years since you've really connected, but she will let you know. Feel for the energy of this area. Speak with her, tell her: 'I am beautiful, radiant and strong.' 'I am full of passion and creativity.' 'It is safe for me to feel.'

Move with her by sending warm orange light to the area around your hips and the centre of your belly below your navel. As this area is the centre of your sensuality, moving with the tune of your body will awaken the senses 'down there'. Put on some sensual music and move your hips — keep it slow, listen to how she wants to move. She is the Divine Feminine and so are you.

Shame and blame

While we may live in a sexually liberated world, many of us have NO idea as to who we are as a sexual woman. Many of us are simply following a story of how we *think* it should look and feel, thanks to the mixed messages we receive from the media and pornography, but how do we *really* feel? I know personally, I felt shame for the longest time, but couldn't figure out why. For lots of women sexual shame is deep seated in a repressive upbringing or in past traumas, but for me, I just couldn't figure it out and this became even more apparent when I met and married the Viking.

Until that point, after years of being in controlling relationships, I was using my sexual power to get what I wanted, but in this relationship there wasn't a power dynamic. I wasn't being controlled and I wasn't *in* control either. Things got pretty interesting for a while as we navigated this new landscape of respect and honouring each other during sex. It was new territory and I didn't have a map.

It was around this time of feeling held, literally and figuratively, by the strong masculine, that I began to allow myself to really explore what it was to be a sexual and powerful woman. As I did so, I found myself getting more and more pissed at the patriarchy for the stories it had made me believe about womanhood and sexuality. Unfortunately for the Viking, he became a representation of patriarchy in male form. I was mad at patriarchy and this made me mad at him. Every time we went to have sex, my vaginal wall would tighten and I'd get furious – at him and at me. There was frustration, LOTS of frustration, and there was anger, shame and embarrassment too. What I know now is that what was happening was actually bigger than just me. It was SHE calling me to heal this wound so that I could heal my mumma's wound, and her mumma's wound.

This was ancestral, and there was centuries of unlearning to do to ease and eradicate the shame of my lineage.

Yet, I thought I was broken.

So many women think they're broken if they don't want sex.

**Guess what? You're not broken,
neither am I – the story we've been
told over and over again about sex
and how it 'should be' is broken.**

Sexual healing

How did I heal? The Viking and I are really good at communicating. We talk all the time. He respects and honours the work of SHE that I do and understands that my teachings and offerings are felt, experiential and need to be fully embodied before I can share. It's not always easy and it's something we work at daily, but both of us knowing where I'm at in my cycle on any given day helps. We also love having sex and talking about sex in and out of the bedroom, so we play. A lot. We both ask for what makes us feel good and we respect each other's wants and desires.

One of my clients recently shared how she didn't want to tell her partner about the work that we were doing together because he'd laugh and make fun of her.

What world are we living in where men have more control over our bodies than we do? Where we're embarrassed to show our bodies love and get informed about how they work? Where we worry as to whether or not our partner will mock us for reading this book or connecting with our vagina, yet they will ultimately want access to our vagina?

I know that I'm blessed to be in a relationship with a dude who gets it, but we really do owe it to ourselves to value, respect and honour our bodies and our lady landscapes because when we do, we attract partners who will support, value, respect and honour us, too.

SHE TRUTH

I speak specifically about the heterosexual experience because that's the relationship I'm in, but what I say here is true of ALL relationships. Honour, respect and value yourself, your body and your sexuality above all things.

Start by asking yourself these questions:

- What's your current relationship with sex?

- Are you tired?

- Are you stressed at work?

- Do you have any health concerns that may be affecting your sex drive?

There could be a million reasons as to why sex isn't fully pleasurable – it may be related to a past sexual trauma or it could be societal or environmental – but sexual healing starts when we're willing to ask questions and get curious about our experience.

You may not realize how significant your past sexual experiences are in how you're showing up in life so, as you expose and uncover your reasons, emotions may make themselves known, the most common being anger and grief. The following exercise can help you move through those feelings and heal.

∼ FEEL IT, RELEASE IT, HEAL IT ∼

Set a 20-minute timer and choose a space where you won't be disturbed or feel conscious that others might see you.

1. Take in three deep womb breaths (see page xxxii).

2. Invite your body to move or create shapes that express how you currently feel when thinking about sex.

3. Are you contracting or expanding? Do you need to be on the ground? What are you feeling and where are you feeling it in your body? Does a particular incident or experience come to mind? Do words or phrases appear?

4. Feel it and express it through moving your body.

5. Write, draw, paint or dance what's coming through; be with it and don't try to escape it. Express it fully in a way that feels good to you.

You may want to continue for longer than 20 minutes, but make sure to end the session with three slow root lock breaths (see page 17) to seal in the healing.

~

Energetic womb imprints

As I described above, everyone you've had a sexual experience with has left an energetic imprint on your lady landscape and sometimes we can stay connected to that person and experience through an energetic cord. Shamanic cord cutting and soul retrieval ceremonies are a powerful way to help release you from the attachment and call back parts of your soul that may unconsciously be connected to them. If during the previous exercise, it became clear that you're still emotionally and energetically connected to a particular person or experience, the following visualization will help you let go.

~ CUTTING THE CORD ~

Find a quiet place where you won't be disturbed.

1. Take three deep womb breaths (see page xxxii) and close your eyes.

2. See yourself standing on a high mountaintop and call in your support squad – SHE/angels/guides/spirit animals to stand

beside and behind you. You are safe, you are supported, you are loved.

3. On a mountaintop in the distance, the person or something representing the experience, stands before you and there is a yellow chord/rope that is connecting you. They can hear you, but they cannot speak or respond to you.

4. Take three deep womb breaths. You are safe, you are supported, you are loved.

5. Tell them all the feelings, emotions and sensations that you experienced at the time and feel right now.

6. When you're finished, take the yellow cord that anchors your womb to them, with your non-dominant hand, and using your dominant hand, cut the cord with your fingers and watch it drop into the space between the mountains. Repeat the following three times: 'I remove all energy that is not mine from my womb space and my physical and energy bodies and I send it back to you.'

7. Place both hand on your womb space in a yoni mudra and welcome in a return to wholeness. Repeat, 'I am whole. I am complete. I am worthy.'

8. Take three deep womb breaths. You are safe, you are supported, you are loved.

9. Afterwards, complete the ritual by smudging yourself with the smoke of sweet grass, sage or Palo Santo, paying special attention to your womb space. Drink lots of water and eat dark chocolate or drink cacao (see page 228).

~

Collect information about what you need to feel safe and satisfied sexually. Don't hand the responsibility of discovering what turns you on over to a lover, take time out to explore and discover what makes you feel good – self-nourishment, masturbation and play are as important to my health and wellbeing as breathing and praying.

What are you doing in your day-to-day life to cultivate pleasure and to turn yourself on? It's important to understand what you need in your environment and from your partner, to feel most safe because then you'll be open to receiving the very best kind of pleasure – and that's the main goal here. If you become aware of sexual challenges, take time out of relationships to do some self-exploration.

Before I met The Viking, I was on a six-month boyfriend detox. I consciously took time out to be celibate and give myself time to realign with myself and my needs. I read a LOT of erotica – that seriously gets me off. *The Delta of Venus* by Anaïs Nin is HOT (*actually anything by Anaïs Nin is hot*).

Self-nourishment

I think this is my favourite of all SHE Flow practices, as it's when we get to work out *exactly* what we want and desire. You cannot expect others to give you pleasure if you don't take ownership of your body and become the sensual, sexual, spiritual authority on your orgasms, your vagina, your entire lady landscape. If you explore, connect and understand your body, you can tell someone else what you love, what you desire, what feels good and what's a hell freakin' no.

The focus on orgasm/coming/releasing being the main reason to have sex is masculine in its nature. Women are lucky, we are multi-orgasmic, and we begin to orgasm from the moment we're first stroked or touched in a way that feels good. Oh yeah.

Vibrators can be a reliable and fun way to explore what turns you on but rather than chasing an end result, you might like to enjoy simpler ways of exploring pleasure and feeling aroused. Before you reach for the technology, try this simple exercise in self-love.

~ EXPLORING PLEASURE ~

Before starting you might like to put on some music that makes you feel sexy, dim the lights and get comfortable.

1. Take a deep breath. On the exhale, slowly begin to gently rub and stroke every part of your body. Not in the way a massage therapist would, but like you're running your fingers over a lover you adore. Start by rubbing each hand, each finger, each wrist; stroke your fingers across your throat, really allow yourself to explore your body.

2. Find the places that feel good, the sensations that make you groan a little and send love to your body through your touch. This will feel different in each phase of your menstrual cycle, so become curious of your body's need for touch in each phase. So many of us wake in the morning and scan our body for what doesn't feel good – it never occurs to us instead to explore what feels really GOOD. Touch your hands, arms, fingers; stroke your face, your lips, your belly, your yoni, your legs; do what feels good. Don't avoid the areas that you don't appreciate. In fact, pay them more attention.

3. Stroke your yoni.

4. Trace your labia lips with a finger, give gratitude and big love with each stroke – give love and thanks for your body, to SHE, as you stroke and touch her.

So many of us pay no attention to what our yoni loves unless someone is having sex with us. Take back your power and do this exercise regularly, daily if possible. Add positive mantras such as, 'I am powerful' and 'I love my pussy' as you do it. Make it as decadent and as love-filled as possible.

You might also like to read *Autobiography of an Orgasm* by Betsy Blankenbaker – it's her story and devotion to self-healing through orgasm that inspired this practice. The woman is fearless in her sharing and I love her for it.

~

Yoni eggs

A healing practice that I discovered during my boyfriend detox was inserting a crystal egg into my vagina. (*I know, right?!*)

At one time, yoni eggs were simply known as jade eggs, and their use has been traced all the way back to China over 4,000 years ago. At that time, jade was considered a super expensive stone reserved only for women in the royal household who would use jade eggs to tone and strengthen their yoni for general health and sexual prowess. Jade is used predominantly as it releases negative thoughts, soothes and calms the nervous system, and stimulates ideas.

More recently – with the global accessibility of various stones and crystals – other stones are now used too, including:

- Obsidian – weightier than jade and provides insight. (I'm currently working with an obsidian egg and it has been super powerful in helping me to understand the cause of my endo-metriosis and PCOS symptoms, and facilitating my mumma line ancestral healing.)

- Aventurine – promotes compassion, empathy and enhances creativity; calms anger and irritability and balances masculine and feminine energy.

- Rhodonite – assists emotional healing, stimulates, clears and activates the heart chakra.

Why use a yoni egg?

Hectic lifestyles, stress, genetics, pelvic injuries, childbirth, weight loss, weight gain and bad posture can all impact the strength of our pelvic floor muscles, which is why everyone can benefit from a yoni egg practice in every phase of their lives. In our early 20s it helps us to understand and connect with our yoni, it increases blood circulation and vitality to the uterus, ovaries, cervix and pelvic floor, and tones and strengthens the vaginal walls. After childbirth it can help tone up the vaginal muscles that have worked so hard during pregnancy and labour. In our menopausal years, the egg can also help with hormonal balancing by increasing oestrogen.

SHE TRUTH

Don't use a yoni egg during pregnancy or if you have an IUD fitted.

There are many energetic and spiritual benefits to connecting deeply with your yoni using a crystal egg. I've described how many of us feel a sense of shame and disconnect when it comes to our yoni but as you work with your egg in a conscious and delicious way – you begin to heal these things – pleasurably.

I asked my go-to girl for jade/yoni eggs, Jillian Anderson at earthbodymama.squarespace.com, to share why she loves her jade egg practice and why you'll love yours, too.

MUFF MUSE - JILLIAN ANDERSON

If you want to reclaim your pleasure and embrace your desires, starting a jade egg practice will be your new medicine. In fact, there are 21 incredible reasons to start a yoni egg practice:

1. *To tone, strengthen and balance the pelvic floor muscles*

2. *To increase cervical fluid*

3. *To increase fertility naturally*

4. *To alleviate pelvic floor pain*

5. *To balance the left and right quadrants of the pelvic floor (feminine and masculine)*

6. *To reconnect to your sexuality*

7. *To increase libido*

8. *Increase pleasure and sensation*

9. *To stop your partner from ejaculation or bring him to climax (your call)*

10. *To enhance creativity and power*

11. To heal past sexual trauma

12. To release stagnant energy from the pelvis

13. To reduce/eliminate PMT

14. To reduce/eliminate painful menstruation

15. To promote hormonal balance and harmony

16. To increase power, frequency, and duration of orgasms

17. To encourage deeper awareness and articulation of the vaginal muscles

18. To encourage healing dreams

19. To assist postpartum healing/recovery

20. To assist birth trauma healing

21. To prevent/remedy incontinence

My own jade egg practice has led me from one breakthrough to another. Since beginning I've become much more orgasmic. I can do things with my lady parts that I didn't even know were possible (like spin my egg clockwise internally). I can honour my feminine side and trust her inner knowing, and I can feel my sense of self-worth continuously blossoming to new levels.

I now look at the girl I was and see that she lacked a sexually embodied female guide-ess. My primary purpose right now is to be that woman. To be wholesome and sexual. To be devoted and orgasmic. To be holy and pleased.

SHE TRUTH

The tissue of your vagina is highly sensitive and absorbent, so make sure you only buy and insert a crystal that's specifically a yoni egg, as other gemstones can often be treated with chemicals or colourings and that may prove ouch-y and NOT healing.

There are many practices you can do with your egg depending on WHY you're using it. Many women buy a yoni egg for sexual reasons so that they can tone and connect with their yoni on a physical level. This is totally valid. However, I'd like to invite you to open your mind (and legs) to the more healing and sensual yoni egg experience.

~ YONI EGG PRACTICE ~

Ideally, start by giving yourself a beautiful and bountiful breast massage (see page 171) before you begin your practice as this will help you not to only connect with your sensual self, but to open and lubricate your vagina, too.

Warm-up

1. Make sure the egg is warm and at body temperature. Place it between your boobs or rest it on your womb space to allow your body to get familiar with it.

2. Begin by spending a few minutes breathing into your womb and right down into the walls of your vagina. Take this time to tune in to yourself and how you're currently feeling. Then lovingly rub and stroke your groin, belly, thighs and vulva.

3. When you feel ready, and holding the larger end of the egg, bring it to your vaginal opening and start to form tiny circles, asking your yoni if she'd like to receive the egg. If she's feeling tight, she may need a little more warming up, but if you get a clear yes, continue.

4. Allow the vagina to yawn open, and gently slip the egg inside. In the beginning, you may need to gently apply pressure on the egg to help it move inside you. Inhale and squeeze the large end of the egg in with your inner labia. On the exhale relax the squeeze and feel your vaginal canal open. This creates a vacuum that will suck in the egg. Smile as you accept the egg into your yoni.

This a practice not a project, so know that over time your yoni will learn to love the egg and draw it in quickly, but have patience. Being able to melt open your vagina is what will open you up to much deeper and more profound pleasure.

Egg-sercise I

1. Lying on your back, place both feet firmly on the floor and bend your knees.

2. Inhale and squeeze your yoni as much as you can, then exhale and relax completely.

3. Repeat five times.

Egg-sercise 2

1. Stay on your back with knees bent and imagine the top of your sacrum is at 12 o'clock, your left hip is at 3 o'clock, your tailbone is at 6 o'clock and your right hip is at 9 o'clock.

2. Slowly press the top of your hips down to the floor and gently roll towards the left, 3 o'clock. Keep rolling towards your tailbone, 6 o'clock, towards the right, 9 o'clock, and then back to 12 o'clock.

3. Slowly continue to move around in this sensual circle six times. Then go in the opposite direction six times.

Egg-sercise 3

1. This egg-sercise is designed to help you start noticing the subtleties and building up strength.

2. In the same position as egg-sercises 1 and 2, inhale, and press your pelvis high up off the floor, applying the root lock (see page 17) as you do. Now, exhale and relax fully as you roll down vertebrae by vertebrae. Repeat nine times.

3. Now lie on your back, legs outstretched, and surrender. Scan your body for any shifts in your physical, emotional and spiritual body.

Taking out your yoni egg

I panicked when my yoni egg didn't come out the first time, which obviously caused my vaginal walls to tighten and create a super-firm grip on the egg. Cut to my overactive imagination thinking up all the ways to explain why I have a crystal egg in my vagina to the nurse in A&E (ER).

The easiest way to take out your egg is to lie down, take some deep womb breaths (see page xxxii), relax and then push. If your egg has a string you can give it a gentle pull or come into a squat and push the egg out. If this doesn't work – don't panic – just relax and she'll tell you when she's ready to let it go.

How to look after your egg

I treat mine like a sacred item and wrap it in red cloth and keep it on my altar when I'm not using it. After your practice, simply rinse it with warm water, making sure to clean the drilled hole (a pipe cleaner works well) and then wrap it up ready for next time.

At each full moon I put her out for a lunar-boosting energy uplift.

~

Yoni heal and release

When I was experiencing trouble reaching orgasm, I was recommended a yoni massage. Yep, there are practitioners who specialize in internal vaginal massage as a way of helping women overcome sexual trauma or lack of orgasms and they're super skilled in providing touch and techniques that really help to create a safe space in the yoni. I booked an appointment, but I'll be honest, I rang and cancelled at the last minute. Not because I was embarrassed, but because I really wanted to put my own teachings into action and learn to trust myself by touching myself.

Touching yourself intimately is the ultimate act of radical self-love. It increases your ability to relax, increases the flow of energy to your lady landscape and allows you to build a deliciously personal and trusting relationship with yourself and pleasure.

So what I share here is based on my own experimentation of the teachings I've gathered.

~ YONI MASSAGE ~

How long your yoni massage lasts is entirely up to you, just make sure you create an environment that's sensual and relaxing. So if there's a pile of dirty laundry in the corner of the room, or this morning's cup of tea is still on the window ledge (*please tell me this isn't just me?!*) tidy up, burn a candle/light incense/ spray essential oils and create a soothing environment where you won't be disturbed before you start. And if you've never massaged your yoni before, just remember that it's impossible to do it wrong.

1. Put a rug or on your bed and place a pillow under your hips. Pull your legs into a diamond shape with the soles of your feet together and your knees supported by cushions. Your yoni will now be exposed.

2. Inhale softly through your nose and exhale with a deep 'aahhh' through your mouth. Relax your body and allow any tension to leave your body with every exhale.

3. When your body is totally relaxed, begin to massage your thighs, belly and hips. Touching your lady landscape when you're not aroused or turned on is like diving into a pool of ice-cold water. Not fun.

4. Place warmed grapeseed oil (or an organic lube like YES) on your fingers. Allow your palm to cup your pelvic mound with your fingers lightly placed on your outer labia. Breathe fresh and vital energy into your yoni and exhale stagnant energy out.

5. Begin to stroke the lips of your outer labia, one at a time, squeezing the outer lips steadily between your fingers and sliding them up and down the entire length of the lips. Use soft, relaxed, slow movements. Keep breathing deeply.

6. When you're ready, move to the inner lips and clitoris. These are more delicate and sensitive to touch. Stroke them gently, exhaling any stuck energy.

7. Beginning at the top of your clitoris stroke gently but firmly in tiny circular motions releasing energy and tension.

8. Continue around the entrance of your vagina and massage more firmly around the perineum. Continue to breathe. Don't hold your breath or allow your breathing to become too shallow. Keep breathing down into your yoni.

9. When you return to your clitoris, gently massage the hood back and forth. Stroke her, applying different levels of pressure. Take a finger and rub it down one side of your clitoris and down the other, or if you want more stimulation, then rub directly over her. This is the only organ in your body created solely for your pleasure. Enjoy her, honour her. Revel in her. Try one, two, three and four fingers to stimulate her. What direction is more enjoyable? Up and down? Side to side? Circles? A combination of all three? How much pressure is best?

10. There is no end result, you're not looking to climax (*although if you do, that's amazing – scream, shout and enjoy!*) but allow yourself to simply experience what feels good in your body. When you feel filled up with breath and pleasure, cup your yoni in your palm, send her love and gratitude and gently hold her for five breaths. Exhale a deep pleasurable 'aaaaahhh' at the end.

Practise lots and enjoy!

~

All of the practices I've shared in this chapter are simply a gentle, lubricated finger insertion to guide you into a deeper lady-landscape exploration of your very own and while I'm happy to share, you KNOW this. You've ALWAYS known this.

You are holy AND you are sexual and your body's pleasure should be sought and celebrated.

CHAPTER 8

SHE Tent

*'It is terrible how much has been
forgotten, which is why, I suppose,
remembering seems a holy thing.'*
ANITA DIAMANT, *THE RED TENT*

Welcome to the SHE Tent, ladylove.

If you haven't read *The Red Tent* by Anita Diamant, you NEED to – it should be required reading for every woman. The novel, which describes a sacred space shared by women while they are menstruating, birthing and initiating girls into womanhood tapped a well-spring of longing among modern women. To have a place away from the fast pace of daily life to honour ourselves as sacred would be a welcome relief for most women, especially while menstruating, right?

The SHE Tent is a bit like that – it's metaphorical, so it can be a hotel room, a yurt in the countryside, your bedroom or somewhere you visit for an hour, a day or maybe a whole weekend. You don't have to be bleeding to do it and it can be something you do with friends and sisters or a solo event, whatever you decide. Here is where we remember, reconnect and show reverence for our lady landscape. Where we value and honour our body as a temple. Where we gather healing tools, rest, nap, allow for inspiration, dance, move, breathe.

A SHE puja

In the SHE tent, we hold puja. *Puja* is a Hindu practice in which the devotee shows reverence and devotion to an aspect of the Divine through embodied rituals, invocations, prayers and songs. During a SHE puja, we dive into these rituals and acts to show love and pay homage to the potent and powerful medicine bowl that is the womb-space within the female body. *Jai ma!*

What I share here in the SHE tent is for you to go and explore, play with and delight in.

Allow and receive.

The vagina and womb space is a sponge that has a vast and profound capacity to receive – including that which has been passed down the whole matriarchal line – yeah, basically all of humanity, that's the capacity you have to receive.

So I invite you to take responsibility for your receptive vessel of wonder and allow yourself to play, rest, heal and most importantly, let yourself receive.

Breath

Coming into your body doesn't need anything except breath. Yep, take one breath, and then another. I'm obsessed with breath. I think my husband breathes too loudly (*he doesn't, it's just during my pre-menstrual phase it REALLY feels like it*). I replay my mumma's last breath like a video in my mind daily, and I'm constantly reminded with every inhale and exhale that I missed my dad's last breath. I love listening to my little baby nephew's breath when he sleeps on my chest and I know that when I stop and pay attention to mine, I get out of my head and come into my body.

Breathing, or *pranayama* as it's called in yoga, offers many benefits (*besides keeping you alive, obvs*). Our breath can loosen up muscle tension and when we breathe directly into our medicine bowl, we send vital healing energy to the uterus, ovaries, bladder and cervix. I have a toolkit of breathing techniques which bring me home to my body and self – womb breaths (see page xxxii) root breath (see page 17) and fire breath (see below). This powerful heat-inducing fire breath – while it might not feel very relaxing and rest inducing to do, once you've completed three rounds of fire breaths, make a blanket fort and bask in its warm afterglow – it's SO delicious.

~ FIRE BREATH ~

This breathing technique stimulates all of your metabolic processes, so do this practice in the morning before you eat. You can do it standing, lying down, squatting or crouching on all fours.

It has a very powerful effect on your reproductive organs, so if you have an IUD, don't do it as it may fall out. Don't practise this technique if you're menstruating either.

1. Exhale completely as far as you can, then pull your diaphragm up and under your ribs. Remaining in full exhalation, push the diaphragm strongly down towards your pelvic bowl.

2. Without actively breathing, move the diaphragm up and down so your entire abdomen shakes and ripples. You may possibly feel your uterus and other internal organs as they move.

3. When you can't do this any longer inhale again. Then take equal time to let your breath come and go in its own rhythm.

4. Repeat this 10 times.

5. Take three deep womb breaths (see page xxxii) and then do another round.

~

Rest is radical

All my clients come to me in need of rest.

ALL... OF... THEM...

Mummas, PR girls, even yoga teachers – everyone is rest deprived. Rest is considered indulgent (which is ridiculous, BTW), we feel guilty for 'taking time out' and instead we add extra stress to our already stressed-out life. 'I need to run for an hour today after work,' 'I need to see this friend, go to the dentist, make dinner,' 'I have a to-do list that is never ending.'

We are just not designed to push our bodies to the limit, day after day. Yes, we need to keep active, but if we overdo it at the gym, if we stay late every day at the office, we exhaust our adrenals. Overworking and pushing ourselves depletes us, and leaves us hormonally and emotionally unbalanced, releasing the toxic stress hormone cortisol, which enhances belly fat storage and leaves us suffering from fatigue, insomnia and musculoskeletal breakdown – basically you feel tired, mentally slow and physically vulnerable.

I he second half of your menstrual cycle is a call to come home to yourself, an opportunity to make self-care a priority and allow your body to restore and refuel.

Deep rest and relaxation

Radical Rest is something the Viking and I devised that uses the delicious practice of yoga nidra to drop into deep, deep rest and relaxation. Remember the *Maltese Dreamer* I spoke about earlier? My story about this super curvy goddess is that she's dreaming her life into being through Radical Rest Yoga Nidra. She's my homegirl in reminding me how powerful it is to take time out and receive.

Yoga Nidra is Sanskrit for yogic sleep and is a powerful technique from the Tantra Yoga tradition. It is both the name of a state and of a practice that creates an altered state of consciousness allowing you to relax and heal yourself, expand your imagination, enter the realm of subconscious and super-conscious, effectively manifest seemingly magical changes in your life and clear karmic debris in your life – quite frankly, it's bloody delicious. I use it after every SHE Flow class and workshop, and during SHE Chocolate cacao ceremonies we dedicate an entire half hour to being in this sweet state of rest and natural renewal.

Yoga Nidra works by consciously taking your attention to different parts of the body, which activates the nerves in those areas, this is why it's so good to do after a SHE Flow movement practice because it helps to integrate the impact of the movement into your system. You can also use Yoga Nidra as a portal to SHE – when you're in that deep place of relaxation, insight, downloads and messages can be accessed easily. I often feel like I have direct dial in with SHE when I'm in nidra.

∿ **RADICAL REST: YOGA NIDRA** ∿

Make yourself a comfy nidra nest with cushions and a blanket that you can stay in comfortably for about 30 minutes without moving.

The best way to experience nidra is through headphones. It's not necessary, but it really does enhance the experience. Oh, and a lavender eye mask is really good, too.

Make sure your knees, head and pelvis are supported with cushions and take a deep womb breath (see page xxxii).

There's an instruction video on how to make the perfect nidra nest in the Lady Landscaping Toolkit (see page 251), where you can also download a 20-minute Love Your Lady Landscape nidra. Put it onto your music device, put on a pair of over-ear headphones (they're so much better for nidra) and allow your body to fully surrender to the practice of Radical Rest. Deep sigh.

Have some dark chocolate or cacao (see the recipe on page 228) available for when your nidra comes to an end. You'll totally thank me for it.

∿

Crystal womb mandala

Andrew Stark is a wisdom keeper of the crystals and is now one of my most treasured and beloved friends. I was struggling with some big mumma grief when I met him and he worked with me to create a crystal womb mandala to help me heal my personal grief, my matriarchal grief and the grief I'd been holding in my womb space.

So let me explain: a crystal womb mandala is not dissimilar to a crystal grid. A grid is where you combine powerful gemstones with sacred geometry and personal intention, but what Andrew and I created together was a little different. We gathered specific crystals for the purpose of healing womb space, grief and matriarchal patterning, Andrew created a womb grid and then, as I held each crystal in my hand, I placed each crystal on to the grid with this intention: 'I send love and healing to my womb and to my mumma lineage.'

I first worked with my womb mandala in front of my matriarchal rose. The beautiful pink-flowering rose that used to be my nanna's, then when she died my mumma planted it in her garden, and when she died I planted it in mine. I wish on those roses, I cry in front of those roses, I do magic spells with their petals when they drop. I talk to them every morning, but really when I talk to them I'm talking to all the women in my bloodline who are represented by those roses – the women who have shaped me, carried me in their womb, the women who have taught me what it means to be THIS woman in THIS body. So I sat in front of the rose and I began, crystal by crystal to make my mandala.

It was powerful and it was emotional. Really bloody emotional.

Now, some grids are created and then placed in specific places in your house for prosperity, for health, for pleasure and sex – these are some of the grids I have – but this particular womb grid is more of a mandala, because through the meditative action of making it, I'm creating a healing spiral of wholeness directly to my womb. So it's not the kind of crystal grid to keep on an altar (although you absolutely can if you'd like to), it's an energetic practice that I create under the full moon, on my mumma's birthday, on the anniversary of her death and when I want to connect with my matriarchal line.

Together Andrew and I now create magic and love-infused crystal womb mandalas and rituals for clients who are looking to heal past trauma, who wish to understand their womb better, who are experiencing the menopause, and who have had their womb surgically removed and are wanting to connect with their medicine in the potent space that remains.

The crystal womb mandalas are a powerful SHE Flow meditative healing tool, but if you'd like to make your own, you'll find a print-out-able grid that Andrew has designed for you in the Lady Landscaping Toolkit (see page 251).

∼ A CRYSTAL WOMB MANDALA ∼

Print out your womb grid and start by setting an intention. A simple and easy one to begin with would be 'I send love and healing to my womb'.

Choose crystals and stones that are aligned with your intention and that will enhance it. Crystals that are great for womb and reproductive love and health are ukanite, moonstone, celestite, selenite, rose quartz and jasper, but there are no right or wrong stones to use. Choose the ones that you are attracted to. Trust your intuition.

1. Cleanse your space by burning sage or Palo Santo to clear the energy.

2. Write your intention on a piece of paper and place it at the centre of your grid.

3. Start from the outside and work inwards, placing the crystals on the womb grid, trusting your intuition as to what to put where. Feel the healing properties of each crystal in

your hand and keep your intention clear in your mind as you place it down on the grid.

4. When you've finished, take a crystal quartz point or use your finger and, starting from the left ovary, draw an invisible line connecting each stone to the next.

5. When complete, hold your womb space and send her love.

~

Yoni healing steam

Yoni steams are an ancient herbal healing practice that cleanses and nourishes your vagina and womb. (*Yep, totally aware how woo-woo that sounds, but you HAVE read the rest of this book, right?*) When I told Em Tivey from womansoul.co.uk about the dark clotty blood I experience at menstruation — because that's what women who work with periods, womb and all things menstrual talk about when they get together — she recommended I do a yoni steam in my pre-ovulation phase. I'll admit I was sceptical. But Em is a healer and she's my go-to girl for *all* herbal remedies, so I trusted her, tried it and *loved* it. It's now something I do every cycle. My bleed is lighter, I'm less bloated and I have no clots. (*WIN!*)

Traditional midwives and healers in many regions of the world use yoni steam to restore balance in the womb and to treat many reproductive health issues including fibroids, dysmenorrhea (painful menstruation), amenorrhea (absent menstruation), endometriosis and ovarian cysts.

Known in Korea as *chai-yok* and in Spanish as *bajos*, the vaginal steam helps restore health to the womb by increasing warmth, circulation and encouraging a normal menstrual cycle. Quite simply the process of vaginal steaming is basically just sitting over a big cup of herbal tea and soaking it all up!

When to do a yoni steam:

- In the week before your period is due.

- In the weeks after you've given birth.

- After a miscarriage or termination.

When NOT to DO a yoni steam (contraindications)

- If you have an IUD (intrauterine contraceptive device) fitted.

- If you have a fever or infection.

- When you are pregnant.

- When you are menstruating.

- After a caesarean birth (wait for six weeks or until you feel ready).

- Anytime it doesn't feel right for your body – trust your wisdom.

How it works

- Using a blend of organic medicinal plants to make a herbal infusion, the steam rises and opens and lubricates the yoni with gentle healing, cleansing and stimulating properties, supporting a healthy pelvic space and reproductive organs. Vaginal tissue is one of the most absorbent of the entire female body. The steam opens up the pores of the tissues and increases blood flow to the labia and vaginal canal, relaxing the muscular and deep fascia layers of the pelvis and womb.

It warms, soothes and nourishes the internal membranes; provides internal cleansing of the uterus by assisting in the release of incompletely flushed debris, impacted and old endometrial lining. Yoni steams tone the pelvic floor to create a natural healthy lubrication that cleanses, rebalances and restores natural pH level. It also encourages the womb into her natural, open and upright position.

What would you use it for?

Yoni steams are ideal if you have endometriosis, very dark blood or brown fluid (brackish) at the beginning or end of menstruation, irregular periods, painful periods, fertility issues, cervical stenosis, endometriosis, muscle tension/tightness, ovarian cysts, uterine fibroids, prolapsed uterus, pelvic trauma, vaginal dryness or postpartum and post-miscarriage or termination.

How does it work?

Energetically, the steam and herbs are absorbed through the root chakra (see page 182) and pelvic bowl, supporting the release of deep fears and fundamental beliefs that no longer serve you. Herbal steam is akin to the sage smudge that clears negativity and the smoke that carries prayers into the heavens. It allows us to flow into our intuitive being, connect to our wisdom and creative impulse, awakening our wombs and stirring the Shakti within.

What's in it?

You can choose from a variety of herb combinations, but my favourite is a blend of the following:

- **Yarrow herb:** Uterine tonic, pelvic circulatory system stimulant, anti-spasmodic, blood/liver purifying – aura protective and highly healing energy

- **Marigold petals**: Uterine and hormonal tonic, healing tissue, softening scar tissue and adhesions, gentle warmth

- **Rose petals**: Most prized of the womb medicines, soothing, softening, tonic, relaxant, cooling, balancing – aromatic, sensual, loving and nourishing. Total womb loving!

- **Raspberry leaf**: Uterine tonic, nutrient dense, cooling, anti-spasmodic, relaxant –nurturing and protective

- **Sweet violet leaf**: Nourishing tonic to the reproductive system – sacred symbol of abundance and fertility, and like the womb, a holder of the mysteries of life, death and rebirth

MUFF MUSE - EM TIVEY

How to Steam Your Yoni

Heat is medicine for the feminine body. Where cold causes contraction, heat supports opening and release. The moist heat softens the womb and the tissues, increases vital blood flow and supports your womb in releasing any stagnant blood that may have built up.

Set up your steam space; this is a nourishing act of self-care so turn off your phone, put on some music if you'd like to, grab your favourite book, light candles or make a cup of tea to enjoy while you are steaming.

Begin by placing a large handful of the herbs in a large stainless steel pot or bowl with about 9 litres of fresh water on the hob. Gently simmer the herbs in the water for 10 minutes then remove from heat.

Put your bowl under a slotted chair, the toilet seat, a step stool with slats, or if you fancy a work out, you can squat over the bowl, but you will be sitting over the steam for 20 minutes so your legs and bottom need to be comfortable and supported. (You can even make your own steam chair. The Viking made mine by cutting a hole in the seat of a garden chair.)

Get naked from the waist down, cover yourself with a warm blanket or towel that reaches the floor and includes the back of the stool/chair. This creates a 'sweat lodge' over your legs, the chair legs and steam bowl to retain the steam and warmth. It's important to keep your feet warm so wear cosy socks.

Absorb the herbal steam for 20 minutes. If you feel the steam is too hot, remove the bowl and let it cool for a few minutes before resuming.

Rest for at least 30 minutes after the steam to strengthen the healing process and to allow your womb to integrate the effects of the herbal steam.

For a pleasurable bleed and easing menstrual pain, imbalances and blood clots, setting aside time for up to three yoni steam rituals during your pre-menstrual phase is one of the best ways to prepare for your moon time/bleeding phase. The warming steam aids in cleansing and nourishing the uterine membrane. Healthy menstrual blood flows easily, is a bright red colour and has no clots.

For fertility

Yoni steams are a great support in nourishing our lady landscape into a natural state of fertility and creativity by encouraging moist and receptive uterine membranes. If you're actively trying to conceive, you can use the yoni steam during your pre-ovulation phase up until ovulation (see page 90), to prepare for conception but don't steam after possible conception.

After miscarriage

During the vulnerable time following a miscarriage, a yoni steam may support your body in cleansing and can also be a nurturing way to connect with your SHE power centre and avoid pain and trauma taking root in your body. You can begin to yoni steam once your bleeding has ceased. Take the time to honour the initiation of this experience and actively support the energetic and physical release.

Postpartum

Keeping yourself warm is at the heart of many traditional postpartum practices across the world. Using yoni steams after birth brings nourishing heat to your lady landscape, it supports the body to release fluids and aids the womb in shrinking back to pre-pregnancy size. If you have had a caesarean you may want to wait at least six weeks or until you've healed well and fully.

Perimenopause and menopause

When your cycles are slowing down or changing, the yoni steam can stimulate circulation and support your womb to continue to release fully. On the other side of menopause, the warming steam can be revitalizing for vaginal dryness while nourishing a deep connection to your feminine centre and inner woman in a time of initiation and transformation.

Pelvic pain, tightness or pain during intercourse

For women experiencing pelvic pain, chronic holding or tightness, the yoni steam helps to soothe and relax the pelvic muscles. Combine the steam with breath awareness and full deep womb breathing (see page xxxii) to relax your pelvic muscles and create a loving connection with your medicine bowl.

After hysterectomy or pelvic surgery

The heat and warmth can be a soothing therapy for scar tissue. When combined with castor oil packs and massage it helps to increase vitality after surgery. Doing a yoni steam may also be helpful in emotionally and energetically reconnecting with your feminine centre after an invasive procedure and/or experience. Remember your SHE power centre always remains even if you no longer have your physical womb or ovaries.

Castor oil pack

Using a castor oil pack is an easy and effective method to show your womb some love, especially during the pre-menstrual phase of your cycle. It's also a great thing to do after a yoni steam, too. They help break down scarring and adhesions, which are a huge cause of period pain and cramping, and are found commonly in women with endometriosis.

Castor oil is absorbed through your skin and helps to effectively reduce inflammation – it's pretty clever medicine. The Viking is an Ayurveda practitioner and recommends them because the heat helps move stagnant energy, brings fresh, oxygenated and nutrient-rich blood to the womb, and helps to restore the menstrual cycle to a normal balance.

SHE TRUTH

Don't do a castor oil pack while bleeding - either menstruation or irritable bowel syndrome (IBS) - if you're pregnant, if you have an IUD fitted or if you're actively trying to conceive.

~ USING A CASTOR OIL PACK ~

Castor oil packs are great applied after a long bath and you may want to add some essential oils – rose, frankincense and lavender make a really relaxing blend, which is also perfect for calming the nervous system. Oils that have anti-inflammatory properties such as chamomile and lavender are particularly healing.

It's also worth noting that castor oil will stain and can't be removed, so make sure you have a supply of old clothes and towels for the purpose.

1. Warm a few drops of cold-pressed castor oil (available from health food stores) by rubbing it between your palms and then gently massage it into your abdomen area (under your belly button down to your pubic bone, and across to your hips).

2. Lie down with some old towels underneath you. Pour oil into a cupped hand, let the flannel/muslin soak it up and then place onto your womb area.

3. Place a hot water bottle directly over the flannel (you may want to wrap it in an old pillow case so it's not too hot).

4. Once you've got your pack in place, you can kick back and leave it on for about 90 minutes, and really relax. I like to take it to bed with me so I can deeply rest and let it work its magic overnight.

~

Dancing with the Divine

I studied yoga because my belly-dancing teacher said it would strengthen and connect me to my core. She was right, it did do those things and – in strengthening and connecting me to my medicine bowl – it also brought me home.

Movement will always bring you home.

It's why I created SHE Flow yoga. The asana practice of SHE Flow is dance-like in style and doesn't ask you to hold positions for long periods of time – it's inspired by Middle Eastern belly dancing and the classical temple dancers of India. (I am obsessed with temple dancing.)

The Temple Dance of India is based on the tradition of the Deva Dasi, where the dancer consecrates her art as a sacred act for the Divine. The dance becomes a moving meditation of deep devotion and surrender. The dancers convey the epic stories of the gods and goddesses through intricate hand gestures (*mudras*), foot patterns and expression (*abhinaya*) and so the dancer and the dance become one.

I began my journey with Indian temple dance three years ago, and I'm still a total beginner as it takes years of practice, but it has already inspired so much of how I share SHE Flow. Watching the dancers fully surrender to the wild and primal flow of Shakti that pulses through their bodies is IT. You know what that feels like, right? We're told it's when we 'lose ourselves in the moment' but what's really happening is that we're finding ourselves. We're remembering and reconnecting with ourselves and with SHE, and when we do that we become an alchemist, stirring our cauldron and transforming and altering our moods and experience from one state to another.

That's SHE power in action.

Our life is one delicious temple dance to the Divine.

All ancient traditions know this. Wherever you're able to look behind the current patriarchal cycle we're experiencing, you'll find dancing – tribal, fire, ecstatic – all are used to come into communion with SHE in an altered state of feminine consciousness.

Put on your favourite track by a modern-day goddess of your choice and allow SHE to move you through you – there's no right or wrong way to do this. Enjoy the dance! Know that pelvic movements – especially squats – can bring up deep anger, rage and/or grief. If it happens, dare to go there, be with it ALL, it's all part of the dance. This IS SHE Flow.

Dancing is great done alone but is also so good when shared, which is why I have monthly dark moon SHE sessions. At these times, I gather with women and we do SHE Flow together (assisted by cacao) and we experience deep Yoga Nidra, Radical Rest, and we vision quest, nap and share stories.

But most of the time, we just dance. We let our bodies and SHE connect and we dance.

Gather your sisters and g-friends and dance together. Come to a SHE flow class (see Resources, page 247). Attend a belly dance class or Five Rhythms or Qoya – anything that invites you to use movement as a direct way to hook up with SHE and express yourself in all your fullness.

A little known fact about me is that on occasions, I also dance burlesque. My stage name is Gypsy Star Fire and I love how I feel when I dance on stage. I asked my friend Sophia St. Villier, a burlesque dancer and total redheaded goddess, 'What is the connection between the inner goddess and burlesque?'

MUFF MUSE – SOPHIA ST. VILLIER

What I love about burlesque is that it can be anything you want it to be. For me: it's wild, sassy, elegant, silly, glamorous, refined, funny, undomesticated and very, very sexy. Burlesque is an unabashed celebration of the body. In burlesque shows, you see performers enjoying and taking real pleasure in their bodies in public space, something I feel is all too rare. Take tassel twirling with tasselled pasties, for example. It may not be what some people think of as conventionally sexy, but there is a wilderness and power in moving ones body with such aplomb, humour and skill. How can that not be seen a sexy?

The big connection between burlesque and embracing my inner goddess for me is that it redefines 'sexy' – on a microcosmic and a macrocosmic level. After burlesque shows and at the classes I teach, I'm often asked 'How can I be sexy?' Or women say to me, 'I wish I was sexy' or 'I'm too (insert put down) to be sexy' – all of which I find heartbreaking. Many of the women who come to my burlesque classes don't necessarily want to jump on stage and perform, but want to embody the confidence and embracement of their own sex appeal in the way that a performer exhibits on stage and then apply these tools in their own lives. I've come to the realization that we have this collective idea of what sexy is and that it is something outside of us – like a club we are excluded from. Yet we don't take the time to define what sexy is for ourselves.

When we do, however, it creates a connection with the Divine. We are seeing ourselves as goddess sees us. A declaration of worthiness, wholeness and don't give a damn-ness. Personally, I think there is nothing sexier and more beautiful than someone smiling from their heart. Just the thought of a smile like that makes my heart feel golden.

There is primal power in sensual movement. Burlesque isn't a standardized dance form, so movements taught vary from one teacher to another. I love teaching old-school burlesque movements like bumps 'n' grinds that bring focus to the second chakra and feel really good to do. If you'd like to try a bump yourself right now, stand up, engage your core (image you are pressing your tummy button to your spine) and swing your hips to the left with a short sharp 'bump' as if you are shutting a car door.

Now bring your hips back to a neutral position and swing out to the right and 'bump' the imaginary car door to your right. If you every come to one of my classes, we do a lot of 'shutting the car door' – ha!

A 'grind' is sensual and raunchy move and best done with a saucy facial expression (as are all burlesque moves). With your legs a smidgen wider than hip width, you are basically going to circle your hips slowly in a big circle over the Mother Earth beneath you.

Try it to Mood Indigo *by David Rose* or Real Gone *by Sam Taylor & His All Star Jazz.*

Menstrual medicine

My nanna, the gypsy witch, and I used to spend a lot of time in the kitchen together when I was a kid making tinctures and get-better potions. When I started my period she'd make me drink a tea for my pre-period and period pain, except I didn't have pain, not then, and she said that was because I drank the tea!

She was totally right, because when she died a year or two after I started menstruating, I stopped drinking it and I got lots of pain, which I turned to pharmaceutical drugs to numb – I bet she's now laughing and saying, 'Ha, Looby Loo', (*that's what she used to call me*) 'I knew you'd come round to my way of thinking eventually – the old ways are the best ways.' I now constantly call on the old ways – her recipes, remedies, spells and tinctures for... well, just about everything.

This gypsy witch brew of raspberry leaf and hibiscus tea is womb healing 101. In herbal healing, red raspberry leaf tea is hailed as a woman's health herb. The claimed benefits range from increasing fertility, toning your uterus, relieving PMT symptoms, such as cramping, irritability, and depression, increasing milk production after pregnancy – it's pretty badass.

The hibiscus flower has been used as an offering to both the Hindu goddess Kali and the god Ganesha and is used in sacred ceremony and ritual in Egypt, Sudan, Hawaii, and by the Dobu of the Western Pacific. It can be found in recipes for moon teas and love potions and in some regions women are banned from drinking it as a tea due to its arousing nature!

Combined, these two herbs are nourishment in a glass and I recommend drinking it in the second half of your cycle to relieve cramps and show yourself love but recently, when exploring cacao as a plant teacher during my pre-menstrual phase, I added Nanna's gypsy tea to Peruvian ceremonial cacao – wowzers! This potent combination is one that I now save for SHE puja and ritual as a devotional offering to SHE.

Nanna's gypsy tea

You will need:

  150ml (5fl oz) hot water

  2 tbsp dried hibiscus flowers

  1 tbsp dried raspberry leaves

  1 pinch ground cinnamon

  1 tsp agave honey (or to taste)

Pour the hot water over the dried ingredients. Leave to steep for 10 minutes and then stir in the agave honey. Breathe, rest and enjoy.

Cacao

I can't talk about radical rest, pre-menstruation and SHE tents and NOT talk about chocolate, can I?

Ixcacao – which literally translates as SHE chocolate – is the goddess of the brown gooey yummy-ness. She's a rich, sexy and abundant Earth Goddess and she is ALL powerful. She's feminine and fierce, and from my experience, working with her will give you what you need, but not necessarily what you think you want.

Every time I enter my pre-menstrual phase, I take her medicine. It's not Cadbury's, it's not processed, it's raw ceremonial cacao and it's bitter. I melt it down, and how I'm feeling will dictate the ingredients I choose to mix with it – sometimes chilli, if I need to evoke some fire, and sometimes coconut milk and honey, if I'm in need of comfort. I then enter into a divinely delicious relationship with SHE, the cacao diva.

The spirit of cacao is a very feminine plant spirit, who works with both the heart and womb. When you work with her, delicious and deep healing and release can take place.

I have often invited the cacao deva to be my creative muse and while writing this, I'm currently undertaking a seven-day cacao diet to connect with my pre-menstrual phase and her needs. I'm drinking cacao as a ceremonial drink and eat a light, plant-based diet for the duration of my pre-menstrual phase because I'm interested in connecting with the rewilding nature of this phase and I want her to hold my hand and guide me as I explore.

I'm trying lots of different recipes but combining Nanna's gypsy tea and Peruvian cacao is by far my most favourite combination and one that I plan on using for every ritual and ceremony. SO GOOD.

Each morning I sit at my altar, drink her in and let her medicine guide me as to what I need to know. Cacao is a powerful facilitator to meditation, yoga, creativity and connection. When I gather women in circle for cacao ceremonies, it's for a four-hour-long, bone-deep nourishing experience. An invitation to enter into a self-devotional practice to meet their wise, wild woman, the one who craves to go deep within, the one who demands personal time away from her family and responsibilities, to fully receive. It's powerful and potent SHE medicine and I LOVE to share it. As Frederick Shilling, author of *Dagoba Chocolate*, says,

**'You can deprive the body,
but the Soul needs chocolate.'**

Did I mention it also tastes REALLY good, too?

SHE cacao

You will need:

> 150ml (5fl oz) hot water
>
> 2 tbsp dried hibiscus flowers
>
> 1 tbsp dried raspberry leaf
>
> 1 pinch ground cinnamon
>
> 57g (2oz) ceremonial cacao, chopped and grated
>
> 1 vanilla pod, deseeded
>
> 1 tsp agave honey (or to taste)

Pour the hot water over the hibiscus flowers, raspberry leaf and cinnamon and then add the cacao. Leave it to steep for 10 minutes or until the cacao has dissolved. Finally add the vanilla and honey. Stir well and enjoy.

LADY LANDSCAPING TOOLS

SHE medicine

- **Touch yourself. Often.** Vibrators are great, but they can desensitize your sexual experience so use your fingers and a great organic lube, and explore, feel and heal your lady landscape.

- **Rest.** Allow yourself to fully lean into the exhale of every breath and take regular time out to breathe, to dance, to She Flow, to drink tea, to eat chocolate instead of feeling guilt or worry about what you 'should' be doing.

- **Love your landscape.** Reclaim your body and retell your story in a way that feels real, nourishing, true and nurturing to you.

Mantra

Repeat this mantra any time you need a reminder:

'I am open to receive.'

#BLOODYCONVERSATION STARTERS

These can be used as journal prompts, dive-deeper questions, book club or SHE circle themes or, y'know actual bloody conversation starters on social media, with your g-friends or a stranger on the bus. . .

- Do you have a self-nourishment practice? How do you feel about cultivating one?

- Are you allowing yourself to receive? If not, what's stopping you? The expectation of others? What would it be like if you fully surrendered to the exhale and lived life from THAT place?

- If you showed up whole and in your power, what would happen?

Read

Betsy Blankenbaker, *Autobiography of an Orgasm*

Steve and Vera Bodansky, *Extended Massive Orgasm*

Mantak Chia, *The Multi-Orgasmic Woman*

Anita Diamant, *The Red Tent*

Anodea Judith, *Eastern Body Western Mind*

Anaïs Nin, *The Delta of Venus*

The Whole SHE Bang

'A woman is the full circle. Within her is the power to create, nurture and transform.'
DIANE MARIECHILD

When you remember, reconnect and come into complete reverence for what you knew before you forgot – that your womb is the holy grail and that it's a power portal, oracle and cauldron of healing – you are able to fully access your intuition, your creativity, your connection to source, your innate SHE power.

And it's freakin' amazing.

So that's why I've written this book, to remind you to remember, reconnect and come into reverence, too.

I have spent over a decade on a womb-led SHE quest. I've fully owned words like 'witch' and 'healer' as my truth – despite my matriarchal lineage being fearful of me doing so.

I've visited global sacred sites, received womb blessings and ancient shamanic rites, I've learned the female arts of Mary Magdalene, Isis and the temple priestesses – belly rubbing, blood mysteries, sensual and ecstatic pleasure, the power and ritual of sacred dance and sexual medicine.

I've trained as a menstrual, fertility and reproductive health practitioner, a womb and abdominal massage therapist, a cacao alchemist, a yoga teacher who specializes in lady parts and female bodies.

I still have my womb and ovaries despite the dude-in-the-white-coat's best effort to 'whip it out'. My pain is now virtually nonexistent – hurrah. The only time I suffer is if I let the outside 'noise' of expectations and how I 'should' show up, or need to be 'fixed', become my truth; if my whole expression of being a woman – emotions, anger, pleasure, joy and rage and everything in between – are not recognised/acknowledged/expressed; if I forget/ignore my cyclic nature and slip into old habits of 'doing life like a dude' and over work, over socialize and burn the candles at both ends.

If THIS happens, SHE will be sure to kick me lovingly in the ovaries during my pre-menstrual phase. And guess what? I'm grateful for the reminder. I'm grateful for the continuous invitation to enter into self-enquiry – why's this happening? What am I holding onto? What am I not letting go of? What am I not paying attention to? But most of all, I'm grateful for a built-in map that comes complete with warning signals and superpowers for the terrain that is an authentic, whole and connected woman.

I speak in my outside voice about things that patriarchy has made taboo. I gather with women and invite them to bring it all – their stories, their truth, their anger, their tears, their words, their pissed-off vaginas – ALL of it. (It really shouldn't be a radical act for women to share space in this way, with no structure, no agenda, just an intention to surrender to flow and receive – but it is.)

I've taught and shared lady-landscape healing and created the SHE Flow movement and medicine practice because basically, I'm a lady landscape enthusiast (*ha! I'm totally getting that made into a pin badge*). A woman who wants more than anything for us to rub our third eye and clitoris simultaneously and reconnect, remember, reclaim and be in total reverence for our fierce and feminine SHE power. I'm so ready for a world where we all remember that our truth lies between our thighs, aren't you?

When we remember, we can put ourselves back together again. We grow strong roots, we own our power and we rise. Together.

I want, more than anything, the WHOLE experience.

Not just the Instagram-worthy highlights, but the blood and guts of being a woman – the messy, awesome, passionate, sad, fiery, pleasure-full, anger-filled, badass, ecstatic, painful, hard (*insert word of your choice here*) bits, as well as the awesome bits, the shitty bits and the WTF? bits.

To truly see what patriarchy has had us believe to be true about ourselves and then smash it into pieces. And to keep smashing it until we find the raw energy in the wounds that we've held deep in our wombs and use it to create medicine that supports ourselves, each other and our divine flow as women in the world.

Yeah, I want the whole SHE bang.

The whole SHE bang is when you're able to trust and live from a place of rooted womb wisdom.

It means that sometimes you'll piss people off.

Sometimes you won't receive the outside validation you've been taught to seek and that sometimes you'll feel really bloody lonely.

It means that sometimes you'll cause ripples and other times you'll create earthquakes.

Sometimes you'll be strong and other times you'll need to be held and supported.

Bring it all and love it all.

Love yourself enough to accept and lean into all of what it to be a woman who is wild, sensitive, emotional, intuitive, cyclic and welcome ALL the emotions, feelings, phases and cycles of life, and love it up. Hard.

Welcome yourself home, each and every day. Welcome all the faces and shades of yourself into your womb space and don't leave any part unseen or unloved. The bitch, the aggravator, the manipulator, the lover, the people pleaser – invite them all. Your SHE power will awaken to your willingness to be with ALL of you.

Reclaim your body

It's so important to create a relationship with your body and arrive fully in her every day. This is where you come face to face with SHE and get to REALLY know and own your truth and wisdom. Know that it is safe to be in your body, enjoy being in your body and know that learning to love ALL of your parts is how you call your power back.

Lay your hands on your body, listen to her, dance with her, walk with her, move in SHE Flow with her, say 'it's safe to be in my body' as an affirmation in the mirror each morning, touch yourself, create artwork to honour your yoni. Trust the ways that you feel called to reconnect and enjoy your body.

Love the landscape and terrain
of your body and love the
woman who lives in there.

Drench yourself in pleasure

Forget pressure, it's ALL about the pleasure. We've never been taught that. Pleasure is not something to seek once everything else has been taken care of. Seek it NOW. Splash in it, dance in it, make love in it. Pleasure is necessary.

Let SHE guide you

Let SHE take the lead in your life. Listen to your labia lips, that inner call that says 'do this, go here, I want more of this' and practise speaking, living and acting from THAT truth.

Trust your womb voice. This is your intuition and SHE never lies. It's most accessible in the second half of your menstrual cycle, and if you have trouble hearing her, go for a walk in nature, ask her questions, breathe into her. Then practise giving yourself permission not to have to explain yourself, apologize to, or reason with anyone.

The wisdom, needs, wants, desires and cosmic winks that are SHE-led are the ones that guide you into becoming the woman you REALLY came here to be.

Let your menstrual cycle be your muse

SHE speaks through your body and I've found she communicates most loudly and profoundly through your menstrual cycle. I know it might feel like living in tune with the seasons and our cycles is just not doable in the 21st century, but it's our very nature as women. It's our super power. Most importantly, it's in our blood and it's up to us to reclaim it.

You've only got to watch Mumma Nature flirt with each season and you can see she has it pretty much figured out; she goes with the flow, she follows her instincts, uses what she needs, leaves what she doesn't and begins each day, each season, renewed.

Each month we work lady magic. We are able to access the linear thinking and get-shit-done-ness in the first half of our cycle and in the second half, we come inwards to embody, edit and to cleanse and let go.

When you let your menstrual cycle be your pilot light and muse, you master the courage to believe what you feel and then respond accordingly. You let ancient feminine cyclic wisdom unfurl and become a connecting red thread that guides you deeper into who you truly are. You're a badass, in case you were wondering.

Trust your SHE-scape

How you show up to life on a daily basis is affected by your SHE-scape.

This is the lady landscape, as it looks to you in any given moment, the external and internal weather forecast of being a woman. You can check in with this each and every morning, before you start your day. We live in a linear-dude-centric society, which isn't down with our cyclic nature, and we ARE cyclic.

And when we remember that we're cyclic, when we remember that mumma nature is our mirror, we're able to start remembering and reconnecting with ourselves.

First, know your own stage of womanhood:

- maiden

- creatrix – menstrual years

- wild and wise woman – perimenopause

- wisdom keeper/crone post-menopause

Know it and honour it, sister.

Then check the season outside your window. Is it spring, summer, autumn (fall) or winter? The season that you're experiencing externally WILL impact you internally, so look to eat seasonally and if possible grow your own so you can plant, nourish and harvest in sync with her seasons. Get witch-y and honour the Wheel of the Year, the equinoxes and solstices – the more you connect with Mumma Earth and her cycles, the more powerful your lived experience on the Earth will become.

> *'If we surrendered to Earth's intelligence*
> *we could rise up rooted, like trees.'*
> RAINER MARIA RILKE

Next, know what moon phase you're experiencing. Today, for example, the moon is starting to wane, so we let go of the masculine, straight-line energy we had access to when the moon was waxing and full and today is the day we drop into the feminine half of the lunar cycle – the waning and dark phases.

SHE TRUTH

This crossover day can be a total dick if you don't know it's coming. We're programmed to believe we need to constantly 'do' and produce and show up in EXACTLY the same way that we do indefinitely, but the lunar phases show us that where there's light there's dark. Where's there's waxing, there's always waning.

You can then get super geeky and work out which astrology sign the moon is currently in – I use an app on my phone called 'iluna' (not an affiliate, just love it!), which tells me which phase and which astro sign we're experiencing at any given moment – that's witchcraft RIGHT THERE. If you dig all things astro you may then want to look at what that means for your personal astro chart. (If there's an app for *that*, can you please let me know about it.)

AND THEN! If you bleed, you will be experiencing one of the four menstrual phases:

- pre-ovulation – get shit done

- ovulation – queen of the freakin' universe

- pre-menstruation – charmed and dangerous

- menstruation – go with the flow

And the energy that comes with THAT too.

Phew.

THIS is lady magic.

Knowing your SHEscape will help you to grow roots into the experience of being you. Women's bodies roll with Mumma Nature and the moon, which is why for so much of the time we feel like a square peg in a round hole. Connecting with your SHE-scape will help you to reconnect with yourself and your body so that you are ABLE to let your wild and free nature begin to be felt and fully expressed.

It's been revolutionary for me in those moments when I thought I was freakin' bat-shit crazy.

The good news is, you don't have to have it all figured out right away, it's a practice. There's also nothing wrong. There's NEVER been anything wrong.

As women we are not short of sticks to beat ourselves with. There are the big generic patriarchal/societal ones, there are the ones given to us by partners/family members/work colleagues, and then there are the biggest and most painful sticks of all – the ones that we give ourselves and hit ourselves with repeatedly, on a daily basis.

Right now, you're trying to operate in a world that's totally set up for dudekind – it's goal-driven, clear-cut and consistent, so every time you try to operate within it, you feel instantly bitch slapped with 'I'm not good enough' and 'I'm a failure'.

It's OK to get angry about that. The Viking suggests that anger simply doesn't serve, but do you know what? He, like most of us, has been made to think that an angry woman is dangerous and uncontrollable and while he's not fearful *of* me, he's definitely fearful *for* me, for how an angry woman has been represented in the world. But conscious anger, righteous anger, is the fire that can burn ALL this shit to the ground.

Feel Kali Ma in every cell of your being, put those sticks into the alchemical fire and let all burn.

All. Of. It.

The comparison, the fear of what others think of you, the illusion of what it 'should' be.

All. Of. It.

The number of likes on social media, the fast pace, the linear business models, the thought that seeking pleasure is 'selfish' or 'indulgent'.

All. Of. It.

Burn it ALL to the ground.

It takes work to stay awake to this but your secret weapon is your ability to feel.

To keep connecting to your body and to your emotions – ALL OF THE EMOTIONS – not just the nice ones, but the roll-in-the-mud, raw, dirty, vulnerable, hot and sore emotions and express yourself from THAT place.

Be honest and truthful about how it feels.

Express, emote, show the world your ovaries, sister, and burn, baby, burn. Y'see there's this ancient proverb that says, 'They tried to bury us, but they didn't know we were seeds.' We WERE those seeds and we are now growing roots straight from our wombs, down into Mumma Earth.

We are strong, we are rooted.

Every time you find yourself hating on your body, comparing yourself to a sister, allowing yourself to be separated from your body and each other; every time you think someone is doing better than you are – take a breath, get your bare feet on the earth and plug your toes into the motherboard.

**Re-member the goddess that
they dismembered.**

Root to rise, sister.

Show up in your wholeness. With your child's sick down the front of your shirt, with nothing figured out, with anger, with rage, with questions, without a game face. Because when you show up whole and *re*-membered, it gives another sister permission to show up this way too. When we state our condition in any given moment, when we're honest, when we're not hiding behind carefully curated social media feeds and we let our pussy tell her truth, one by one, we cut the energetic ties that have enslaved us, that have kept us small and that have stopped us from trusting our root wisdom.

Walking/dancing/living a SHE-led path is not easy, it's a constant revealing of the not known and it takes daily root-tending to love your lady landscape, but lady, it's time.

Root to Rise

I want to share the direct download that came from SHE through me while in the Hagar Qim Temple, Malta, and ultimately inspired me to write *Love Your Lady Landscape*:

'I am as old as time. Even older than that.

I hold secrets. So many secrets that I've taken underground.

But I will rise. I will rise with power. Not brute force, but rooted strength – I will pull down energy from the sky, from the stars, I will pull up energy from the earth and I will rise up through you.

I will be strong in you.

I ask you to simply be open to receive.

To allow yourself to be fully charged with SHE.

Rest.

Dream.

Move.

Sweat.

Cry.

Dance.

Allow and receive it all.

You will have to challenge beliefs and perceptions – those of others, but mostly your own – when you feel resistance, when you feel challenged, place both feet on Mumma Earth and breathe. Breathe deep.

Allow yourself to trust that you know.

You know exactly what needs to happen next.

You know exactly what's being asked of you.

You know exactly what you need to remember for ALL our sakes.

Trust yourself.

Trust what you feel to be true.

Are you ready?

Please say you're ready.

Trust your womb.

Root to rise.

It's been far too long and I'm getting cranky down here.'

We are ALL Called Girls. This is our call.

Closing SHE Ceremony

The candle is still burning as our time together in ceremony is now coming to a close. I invite you to shake, circle and move your body before allowing yourself to find stillness either sitting or standing with your palms facing upwards.

Imagine your entire lineage of women standing behind you, going all the way back to the very beginning. See each of them all holding on to a piece of red thread and then imagine your mumma in pure love, wrapping the red thread around your waist and hear her, and all the g-mummas who have gone before you, say:

> 'We love you, we love the woman that you are, we honour and recognize your power. It's safe for you to be seen and for your voice to be heard. You have everything you need in your womb space. You are love, you are lovable and you are loved. We've got you.'

Take a big deep womb breath.

Now honour yourself.

'I love the woman I am. I honour and recognize my power. It's safe for me to be seen and for my voice to be heard. I have everything I need within my womb space. I am love, I am lovable, I am loved. I've got this.'

Take in another deep womb breath and allow that breath to grow roots from your womb through your thighs, down into your feet and out through each toe into the motherboard.

You are a woman unto herself. You are love, you are lovable, you are loved.

And... So... It... Is...

I LOVE MY LADY LANDSCAPE

For those times when you need reminding, rip this page out or, if like me the idea of ripping a page out of a book gives you the full body chills - and not in a good way - photocopy it, scan it, write it out in your best handwriting, stick it to your computer, on your bathroom mirror, in your journal, make a meme and put it on social media or put your hand over it and say it like a prayer, because. . . well, it kinda is.

- Value your vagina.

- Drink water.

- Go on womb-led adventures.

- Write your own story.

- Dare to share what's true for you. (And never be afraid to change your mind.)

- Trust your body's wisdom.

- Take up space.

- Own your cyclic super powers and use them for good.

- Don't be afraid to get angry. Conscious anger is necessary.

- Touch yourself. Often.

- Know that if it's not a 'hell yes', it's a no.
  Act accordingly.

- Take regular dance breaks.

- Know that your ovaries are thunderbolts of lady magic.

- Honour SHE.

- Love hard.

- Bleed on it.

- Root to rise.

- Avoid douchebags (both kinds).

Resources

The SASSY SHE

thesassyshe.com is fierce and feminine, moon and menstrual-led ancient wisdom made accessible, relevant, devotional and fun for women navigating a modern world.

The SASSY SHE is dedicated to helping you crack your lady code using SHE Flow — yoga, sacred movement and ancient menstrual health practices, rituals and ceremonies — to access monthly super powers that can be used to create a bloody amazing life. Period.

If you've loved what you've read in this book and want to go deeper, you can experience SHE Flow through online programmes, one-to-one mentoring, online classes, workshops and retreats.

Healing and wellbeing for your lady parts

womansoul.co.uk for yoni steam herbs with detailed instructions on how to use them from the amazing Em Tivey.

fertilitymassage.co.uk for massage therapy that brings harmony and balance to the reproductive, digestive and sacral areas.

earthbodymama.squarespace.com for feminine planetary healing.

Lady landscape insight

beautifulcervix.com celebrates the beauty and intricacies of women's bodies and fertility.

thelunarwomb.com invites you to experience the lunar cycle as a dynamic relationship with the moon that is unique to YOU.

theriteofthewomb.com introduces the 13th rite of the Munay-Ki and lets you know where your nearest womb keeper is. If you're in the UK, I offer the rite at every Red Reconnection (see page 123) and SHE Flow workshop (see page 247).

mymoontime.com is an amazing app that tracks your female energy potential.

daysy.me for a fertility monitor and ovulation calculator. My chosen alternative to hormone contraception.

Bloody brilliant eco-friendly menstrual products

honouryourflow.co.uk

holysponge.net

gladrags.com

lunapads.com

moontimes.co.uk

Lady landscape loves

jessgrippo.com is a New York-based creativity and dance coach and tutu-wearing badass.

theherosoul.com for fire-walking experiences with Lisa and Rich Lister.

facebook.com/thecrystalstudios for amazing, high-quality and great-value crystal goodness and my partner in crystal womb mandala creation.

Love Your Lady Landscape: Let the Exploration Begin

My big wish is that this book is the first pussy stroke of a lifelong adventure with your lady landscape. Here are some ways to help you navigate and explore the terrain further:

loveyourladylandscape.com

Meet the muff muses, download playlists and SHE Flow practices, and visit the shop for organic lube, handheld mirrors and plush vulvas. *Oh yeah.* You'll also find details of Love Your Lady Landscape/SHE Power classes, workshops and temple retreats, too.

Lady Landscaping Tools

Throughout the book I share a LOT of breath, movement and nidra practices, so I've put together a free downloadable tool kit of instruction videos and print out sheets – and yep, there is a colour-in vagina to download, too. What's not to love about that?

SHE Power - the online course

If what you've read has you craving more lady landscape love, then you are going to LOVE the SHE Power course, a 28-day online muff dive/immersion that will guide you to find gratitude, reverence and fierce love for your womb, your body and your power.

#loveyourladylandscape

Share the lady landscape love – I'd love to see you reading the book, creating yoni art or colouring in your vagina – by using the hashtag #loveyourladylandscape on social media.

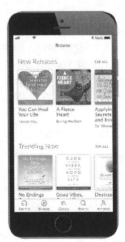

ABOUT THE AUTHOR

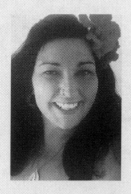

Lisa Lister is a SHE-led menstrual maven dedicated to helping women crack their lady code and love their lady parts.

Lisa's a third-generation gypsy witch and the founder of SHE Flow – a personal invite for women to celebrate the fiercely feminine, sensual pleasure of being a woman through movement, massage, menstrual mysteries and magic.

She's a called girl (not to be confused with a call girl, that's something entirely different) – a called girl experiences life moment to moment. She doesn't hold on too tightly to a defined and specific outcome, in fact she doesn't much care for that at all. Instead she shows up, raises her heart and boobs to the sun, open to the infinite possibilities that occur when you collaborate with SHE – the divine/goddess/universe/spiritual homegirl – to make epic shit happen.

Lisa is doing a lifelong edge-walk with SHE, and through the moon, menstrual and Mumma Earth cycle wisdom, she calls you to walk, dance and roar with her there too.

She also has great tattoos, piercings and a fabulous ability to accessorize.

 @sassylisalister

thesassyshe.com
loveyourladylandscape.com

HAY HOUSE

Look within

Join the conversation about latest products,
events, exclusive offers and more.

  Hay House UK

  @HayHouseUK

  @hayhouseuk

♥ healyourlife.com

We'd love to hear from you!

Printed in the United States
by Baker & Taylor Publisher Services